Premature No More: Simple and Natural Home Remedies to Combat Premature Ejaculation for Improved Performance

By

Patti W. Nieves

Disclaimer:
This book is intended for informational purposes only and is not intended to provide medical advice or diagnosis. The information presented in this book is based on the author's personal experiences and research and should not be considered a substitute for professional medical advice, diagnosis, or treatment. Always seek the advice of your physician or other qualified healthcare provider with any questions you may have regarding a medical condition. The author and publisher disclaim any liability or responsibility for any adverse consequences resulting directly or indirectly from the use of information contained in this book.

About the Author

Patti W. Nieves is a passionate advocate for sexual well-being and pleasure, dedicated to empowering individuals to embrace their sexuality and cultivate fulfilling intimate relationships. With a background as an experienced content creator, Patti has spent years researching, writing, and educating others on topics related to sexual health and wellness. Driven by a desire to break down stigmas and barriers surrounding sexual issues, Patti brings a compassionate and nonjudgmental approach to her work. Through her writing, she strives to provide accessible and inclusive information that promotes understanding, acceptance, and empowerment.

Patti's commitment to sexual well-being extends beyond her professional endeavours; she is deeply invested in supporting individuals on their journey towards greater intimacy and satisfaction. With a focus on holistic approaches and natural remedies, Patti offers practical insights and actionable strategies to help readers overcome challenges and unlock their full sexual potential.As an advocate for sexual well-being and pleasure, Patti believes that everyone deserves to experience joy and fulfilment in their intimate lives. Through her work, she aims to inspire individuals to explore their desires, communicate openly with their partners, and embrace a life of sexual vitality and connection.

Table of Contents

Introduction:

In the dance of intimacy, premature ejaculation can sometimes feel like an unwanted curtain call, cutting short the show before it hits its crescendo. But fear not, for in the world of natural remedies lies a symphony of solutions ready to harmonise with your wishes.

Picture this: You and your partner, bathed in the soft glow of candlelight, ready to start on a trip of desire and pleasure. Yet, just as the beat begins to build, premature ejaculation throws a discordant note into the song, leaving both partners eager for an encore.

But worry not, for within these pages, we open the secrets to extend your performance, allowing you to take centre stage with confidence and vigour. Gone are the days of fleeting moments and failed expectations – welcome to a world where natural solutions reign supreme, and men retake their proper place as masters of the bedroom.

Join us as we dive into the depths of premature ejaculation, discovering its nuances and exploring the transformative power of simple, natural remedies. Together, we'll rewrite the story of closeness, creating a tale of prolonged pleasure and boundless joy. So, without further ado, let us start on this trip towards a future where premature is but a faraway memory, and every moment is a symphony of joy.

Prepare to start on a journey where the peak isn't just a brief moment but a crescendo of pleasure, where each touch stays and every feeling is savoured. Here, in the world of natural medicines, we accept simplicity as the cornerstone of our quest for control over premature ejaculation.

Gone are the days of depending solely on fleeting answers or difficult measures. Instead, we accept the knowledge of nature, tapping into its wealth to nourish both body and soul. No potions or elixirs offering miraculous changes, but rather gentle nudges towards balance and harmony.

But why, you might wonder, place our faith in nature's embrace? Because within its embrace lies an ageless knowledge, a symphony of elements perfectly orchestrated to support and heal. Here, in the simplicity of herbal medicines and holistic practices, lies the promise of permanent change.

In the fabric of human experience, our sexuality is a vibrant thread that weaves together emotion, closeness, and satisfaction. Yet, for many men, the threat of premature ejaculation puts a shadow over this tapestry, robbing them of the fullness of their sexual expression.

But fear not, for within the folds of nature's hug lie the keys to unlock a world of prolonged pleasure and improved performance. In this guide, we'll start on a journey of discovery, exploring the simple yet powerful home treatments that can change premature ejaculation from a hurdle into a chance for growth and connection.

Imagine a future where every personal meeting is a symphony of feeling, where time seems to stand still as you bask in the ecstasy of the moment. This is not a faraway dream but a physical reality within your grasp, ready to be unlocked through the gentle alchemy of natural remedies.

So, dear reader, let us put away the shackles of doubt and limitation, and accept the boundless potential that lies within each of us. Together, let's retake our proper place as stewards of our own happiness, architects of our own satisfaction.

As we start on this transformative path, let's stop to recognize the courage it takes to face challenges and seek solutions. Premature ejaculation is not merely a physical event but a highly personal experience that can impact self-esteem, relationships, and general well-being.

In the hustle and bustle of modern life, it's easy to feel swamped by the myriad of solutions offering quick fixes. Yet, amidst the noise, it's the gentle whispers of nature's remedies that often echo the strongest. In simplicity lies power, and in natural remedies lies the potential for deep healing and change.

So, whether you're here seeking relief from the grip of premature ejaculation or simply curious about overall ways to men's performance, know that you've come to the right place. Within these pages, we'll explore a tapestry of natural remedies, lifestyle changes, and practical methods meant to strengthen you on your journey towards prolonged pleasure and improved closeness.

Together, let's accept the beauty of simplicity and the power of nature's bounty. Let's chart a path towards a future where premature ejaculation is not a barrier but a stepping stone towards greater self-awareness, resilience, and satisfaction.

Premature Ejaculation: A Brief Exploration

Picture this: You're on a rollercoaster ride of pleasure, rising through the peaks of intimacy, when suddenly, the journey comes to an abrupt stop. Premature ejaculation, often described as the premature coming of the grand finale, is like hitting fast forward on a movie reel before the story has a chance to unfold.

In simple words, premature ejaculation is when a man reaches climax and ejaculates sooner than he or his partner would like during sexual action. It's like blowing out the candles on your birthday cake before you've even made a wish – annoying, to say the least.

But why does it happen? Well, sometimes it's like your body's internal clock is set to snooze mode, causing ejaculation sooner than expected. Other times, it's like a race car revving its engine a bit too excitedly, speeding towards the finish line before the race has even started.

Premature ejaculation can leave both lovers feeling unsatisfied and can put a damper on the dance of closeness. But fear not, for there are ways to hit the pause button, allowing you to extend the pleasure and savour each moment like a fine wine.

So, whether you're a seasoned lover or just dipping your toes into the waters of closeness, understanding premature ejaculation is the first step towards reclaiming control and changing the story of your sexual experience.

Think of premature ejaculation as the overeager friend at a party who comes too early and leaves everyone feeling a bit awkward. It's like trying to enjoy a fine meal when the dessert comes before the appetiser.

But here's the thing: premature ejaculation is incredibly common and nothing to be ashamed of. It's like a hiccup in the beat of closeness, a speed bump on the road to pleasure. And just like any hiccup, it's something that can be handled and solved with the right method.

Imagine it as a cunning imp, playing tricks on your time and leaving you scratching your head in frustration. It's like trying to answer a puzzle with missing pieces, leaving you feeling puzzled and unsure.

But fear not, for within these pages, we'll solve the mysteries of premature ejaculation and discover the keys to unlocking a world of prolonged pleasure and happiness. It's like finding the missing puzzle parts and finally seeing the whole picture come together in perfect balance.

So, whether you're a seasoned navigator of intimacy or a newbie to the world of pleasure, know that premature ejaculation is just a temporary detour on the journey towards greater satisfaction. With a little understanding and the right tools in your toolbox, you'll soon be back on track, navigating the seas of love with confidence and grace.

The Importance of Natural Remedies for Men's Performance

Picture this: a lush yard where every plant, every flower, every leaf holds the key to health and well-being. In this garden, nature's medicines grow abundantly, giving a gentle yet strong option to synthetic solutions. Now, imagine harnessing the power of this natural bounty to improve men's ability in the bedroom.

Natural medicines are like the guards of our health, holding firm against the tide of artificial substances and chemical concoctions. They offer a haven of simplicity, a hideaway where purity reigns supreme.

When it comes to men's performance, natural remedies play a vital part in supporting the body, mind, and spirit. They're like the gentle whispers of knowledge passed down through generations, telling us to honour the innate intelligence of our bodies.

Unlike their synthetic rivals, natural medicines work in harmony with the body's natural rhythms, gently pushing it towards balance and vigour. They're like the gentle caress of a breeze

on a summer's day, soothing and invigorating all
at once.

But perhaps the true beauty of natural medicines
comes in their accessibility. They're like jewels
waiting to be found in the depths of the earth,
ready to be unearthed by those willing to listen
to nature's whispers.

In the area of men's performance, natural
remedies offer a beacon of hope for those
looking for alternatives to standard methods.
They're like the guiding stars in a dark sky,
lighting the way towards greater intimacy,
pleasure, and happiness.

So, whether it's herbal supplements, food
changes, or mindfulness practices, let us accept
the power of nature's cures and start on a
journey towards overall well-being. After all, in a
world filled with complexity and noise,
sometimes the simplest answers are the most
deep.

Imagine natural medicines as the strong base
upon which we build our journey towards
improved vigour and happiness.

First and foremost, natural treatments offer a gentle approach to handling men's performance issues. Unlike harsh chemicals or invasive procedures, they work in balance with the body's natural processes, honouring its inner knowledge and equilibrium. It's like giving the body a gentle nudge in the right way, allowing it to find its own road towards balance and vitality.

Moreover, natural treatments often come with fewer side effects and risks compared to their synthetic peers. They're like a soothing balm for the body, giving relief without the added load of unwanted effects. This makes them particularly attractive for those who prefer a more holistic and sustainable approach to health.

Another key feature of natural medicines is their accessibility. From herbal supplements to food changes to awareness practices, these treatments are easily available to anyone willing to explore them. It's like having a treasure trove of health tools at your fingertips, just ready to be found and utilised.

But perhaps the most convincing reason to adopt natural remedies for men's performance is their ability to create a deeper relationship with oneself and one's partner. By honouring the body's natural rhythms and nurturing its vigour, these treatments pave the way for greater closeness, pleasure, and happiness. They're like the threads that weave together the cloth of our most personal moments, strengthening the ties of love and connection.

In sum, natural treatments are not just about solving surface-level concerns; they're about fostering holistic well-being and reclaiming control over our sexual health and vigour. So, let us accept the power of nature's cures and start on a journey towards a future where men's performance is not just about endurance, but about embracing the fullness of our sexual selves.

As we journey further into the world of natural treatments for men's performance, let's explore their significance in encouraging long-term health and vigour.

Another amazing aspect of natural remedies is their ability to address the root causes of performance problems, rather than simply masking symptoms. They're like spies, finding the underlying imbalances or deficiencies that may be adding to problems like premature ejaculation or erectile dysfunction. By addressing these root causes, natural remedies offer the potential for lasting change and sustainable growth.

Furthermore, natural remedies often support general health and well-being, stretching far beyond the world of sexual performance. For example, dietary changes aimed at supporting hormonal balance or lowering inflammation can have significant effects on both physical and mental health. Similarly, techniques like mindfulness and stress management not only improve sexual performance but also promote relaxation, resilience, and emotional closeness.

In a world inundated with quick fixes and instant satisfaction, natural remedies remind us to develop patience and trust in the body's organic healing potential. They're like seeds placed in rich soil, requiring time, nurturing, and patience to blossom into bright expressions of vitality.

Moreover, natural remedies empower people to take an active part in their own health and well-being. They're like the compass guiding us towards self-discovery and strength, encouraging us to listen to our bodies, honour our instincts, and make educated choices that fit with our values and goals.

Finally, natural remedies for men's performance offer not just a means to an end but a pathway to overall health and vigour. They're like the gentle breeze that whispers of possibility, asking us to accept our natural potential and reclaim our vitality, one step at a time. So, let us start on this trip with open hearts and open minds, trusting in the wisdom of nature to guide us towards a future filled with vitality, happiness, and satisfaction.

Join us on this changing journey as we'll unravel the mysteries of premature ejaculation and discover the keys to unlocking a world of prolonged pleasure and happiness. A trip towards a future where premature ejaculation is but a distant memory, and every moment is a call to enjoy the sweet nectar of love and connection

Welcome, dear reader, to "Premature No More: Simple And Natural Home Remedies to Combat Premature Ejaculation for Improved Performance." Here's to regaining our sexual energy, one gentle remedy at a time.

Chapter One:

Unlocking the Mystery Behind Premature Ejaculation: A Journey of Discovery

Welcome to the gateway of understanding, where we untangle the mystery of premature ejaculation and shed light on its complex tapestry. Imagine this as a map, leading you through the maze of premature ejaculation with clarity and kindness.

In this chapter, we start on a quest to decode the essence of premature ejaculation, peeling back the layers to show its true nature and effect. It's like entering a poorly lit room, armed with a lantern of information to reveal the shadows of misconception and confusion.

So, prepare to start on a trip of discovery, where each revelation brings us closer to unravelling the secrets of premature ejaculation. Let's throw away the cloak of stigma and misinformation and start on a quest for truth and knowledge.

As we dig deeper into the realm of premature ejaculation, let's start on a quest to uncover its secrets and shed light on its effect. Think of this trip as a voyage into uncharted land, where each step brings us closer to understanding the phenomenon that is premature ejaculation.

Imagine yourself as an adventurer, armed with curiosity and a thirst for information, journeying into the unknown depths of the human experience. Premature ejaculation, like a secret gem buried beneath layers of misconception and misunderstanding, awaits our finding.

But fear not, fellow traveller, for we are armed with the tools of inquiry and understanding to manage this terrain. Together, we'll unravel the threads of premature ejaculation, studying its meaning, deciphering its common causes, and highlighting its effects on both mental and physical well-being.

So, let us start on this journey with open minds and open hearts, ready to challenge myths and misconceptions, and welcome a better understanding of premature ejaculation. For it is through knowledge and kindness that we pave the way towards greater understanding and eventually, towards answers that empower and uplift.

Unveiling the Culprit Behind the Curtain:

Imagine this: You're on a journey of closeness, sailing smoothly towards the shores of pleasure, when suddenly, the trip comes to an unexpected stop. Premature ejaculation, like a mischievous sprite, throws its cloud over the scene, leaving both partners feeling puzzled and unhappy.

But what exactly is Premature Ejaculation? Picture it as the moment when the fireworks go off before the grand finish, stealing the show and leaving everyone asking what happened to the climax. In simple terms, it's when a man drops his magic potion a tad too soon during the dance of closeness.

Now, let's peel back the layers and study the usual causes lurking behind this occurrence. Think of them as the baddies in our story, each with its own unique role in breaking the rhythm of pleasure.

One cause is often performance anxiety, like a dark cloud looming over the scenery of closeness, casting doubt and insecurity. It's like trying to perform a perfect magic trick under the watchful eyes of a sceptical crowd, the pressure rising with each passing moment.

Another common cause is heightened sensitivity, where the senses are like finely-tuned instruments, reacting excitedly to even the slightest touch. It's like walking a tightrope between pleasure and overstimulation, the line between ecstasy and climax fuzzy and uncertain.

But let's not forget the part of biological factors, like hormonal imbalances or neurotransmitter swings, which can throw a wrench into the gears of sexual function. It's like trying to solve a problem with missing pieces, the answer just out of reach despite our best efforts.

So, dear reader, as we explore the maze of premature ejaculation, let us not be daunted by its complexities. Instead, let us welcome the trip with interest and kindness, knowing that understanding is the first step towards freedom.

1. Common Causes of Premature Ejaculation: Unravelling the Mysteries

Premature ejaculation, like a puzzle with missing pieces, can be affected by a variety of factors. Premature ejaculation is often a complicated mix of psychological, biological, social, and medical factors. By understanding these underlying reasons, individuals and couples can start on a journey towards effective control and eventually, better sexual happiness and closeness.

Let's dig deeper into the labyrinth of possible causes, studying each one with interest and compassion.

1. Psychological Factors:

Performance Anxiety:
Performance anxiety is like the shadow that looms over the stage of intimacy, casting doubt and fear onto the players in the story of pleasure. Imagine yourself in the spotlight, every move magnified, every motion examined by an unseen crowd. This is the core of performance anxiety, a psychological barrier that can hinder sexual success and pleasure.

At its core, performance anxiety stems from a fear of judgement and failure. It's like having a big weight on your shoulders, the pressure to perform weighing you down and overshadowing the joy of closeness. Whether it's thinking about satisfying your partner, comparing yourself to past experiences, or fearing embarrassment, performance anxiety can create a self-perpetuating loop of stress and tension.

The mind is a strong conductor, capable of arranging the symphony of happiness or drowning it out with the cacophony of worry. Performance anxiety can hijack this music, upsetting the normal flow of arousal and reaction. It's like trying to dance with lead weights tied to your legs, the freedom of movement suffocated by fear and self-doubt.

Moreover, performance anxiety is often driven by unrealistic standards and social pressures. In a society concerned with performance and perfection, the pressure to shine in every area of life, including the bedroom, can be crushing. It's like following a mirage in the desert, the idea of perfection always just out of reach.

But here's the truth: intimacy is not a show to be reviewed or criticised. It's a dance of connection and openness, a shared journey of discovery and pleasure. By acknowledging and addressing performance anxiety, people and couples can create a safe and loving place where intimacy can grow. It's like dimming the stage and welcoming the freedom to dance in the shadows, knowing that true connection transcends criticism and expectation.

Stress and Anxiety:
Stress and anxiety are like dark clouds gathering on the horizon, throwing a shadow over the scenery of closeness. Picture yourself in the middle of a storm, the winds of worry whipping through the hallways of your mind, and the thunder of anxiety rumbling in the distance. This is the tumultuous territory of stress and anxiety, where the delicate balance of arousal can be disturbed, leaving both partners feeling unsettled and distant.

At its core, stress and anxiety are the body's normal reaction to perceived threats or obstacles. It's like sounding the warning in the face of danger, preparing the body to fight, run, or freeze. However, when this response becomes chronic or intense, it can cause havoc on the delicate balance of arousal and reaction.

Imagine trying to kindle the flames of desire in the middle of a raging storm. The mind becomes preoccupied with fears and concerns, leaving little room for happiness or connection. Stress and nervousness can tighten the muscles, constrict the breath, and raise the heart rate, creating a physiological barrier to closeness.

Moreover, worry and anxiety can undermine confidence and self-esteem, like weeds choking the garden of closeness. Negative thoughts and self-doubt can take root, leading to a vicious loop of fear and performance anxiety. It's like trying to manage a maze with no clear way forward, each twist and turn leading to greater anger and despair.

But here's the silver lining: stress and worry are not insurmountable hurdles. With patience, understanding, and support, people and couples can learn to manage the storms of life with resilience and grace. From mindfulness practices to relaxation techniques to open communication, there are countless strategies for weathering the challenges of stress and anxiety and recovering closeness and connection.

So, let us not be overwhelmed by the storms of worry and anxiety. Instead, let us face them head-on, armed with the knowledge that true closeness transcends the turbulence of the mind, and that love and connection can weather even the strongest of storms.

Relationship Issues:
Relationship issues are like weeds in the field of intimacy, threatening to choke the life out of the delicate flowers of trust and closeness. Picture a lush garden, where the sun's warm rays nurture flowers of love and connection. In this garden, trust and closeness grow, creating a tapestry of love and understanding between lovers.

But amidst this beauty, relationship problems can appear like stubborn weeds, their tendrils reaching deep into the soil of closeness. These problems can take many forms, from communication breaks to unresolved conflicts to feelings of betrayal or neglect. Like weeds in the yard, they fight for resources and attention, diverting energy away from strengthening the ties of love.

Imagine trying to care for a garden overrun by weeds, each one fighting for room and sunshine. Relationship issues can cause a similar sense of overwhelm, leaving both partners feeling drained and discouraged. Trust and closeness, once vibrant and living, can wither in the shadow of unsolved conflict and emotional distance.

Moreover, relationship issues can erode the base of trust that is important for intimacy to grow. It's like trying to build a house on shaky ground, the walls of link weakened by doubt and confusion. Without a strong base of trust, intimacy becomes fragile and subject to collapse.

But here's the thing: just as a skilled gardener can prune away the weeds and nurture new growth, partners can work together to address and settle relationship problems. It takes patience, communication, and a desire to face difficult feelings, but the benefits can be deep.

By nurturing open and honest conversation, learning empathy and understanding, and prioritising the needs of the relationship, partners can create a garden of closeness that is resilient and lively. Trust and intimacy, like delicate flowers, can once again grow under the warm sun of affection, providing a haven of love and connection for both partners to enjoy.

2. Biological Factor:

Hormonal Imbalances:
Hormonal imbalances are like disruptive notes in
the music of sexual function, throwing off the
beat and leaving both partners feeling out of
tune. Picture a symphony orchestra, each
instrument playing its part in perfect rhythm to
create a beautiful tune. In this comparison,
hormones are the conductors, directing the
complex dance of arousal, desire, and reaction.

But when hormones become unbalanced, it's like
a rogue musician stepping onto the stage,
waving their baton out of time with the music.
Hormonal imbalances can develop for a number
of reasons, including age, stress, medical
problems, and lifestyle factors. When this
happens, the delicate balance of hormones that
control sexual function can be altered, leading to
a range of problems, including premature
ejaculation.

Imagine trying to play a piece of music with one
instrument out of tune. No matter how skilled
the players, the end is discordant and
disappointing. Similarly, hormonal changes can
throw off the careful balance of

neurotransmitters and signalling molecules involved in sexual desire and response.

For example, testosterone, often referred to as the "male hormone," plays a key part in controlling libido and sexual activity in men. When amounts of testosterone are too low or too high, it can affect libido, desire, and erectile performance. It's like the bassoon player in the orchestra suddenly playing too loudly or too softly, breaking the balance of the music.

Moreover, hormones like serotonin and dopamine, which are involved in mood control and pleasure, also play a part in sexual function. Imbalances in these neurotransmitters can affect the brain's reaction to sexual stimulation, leading to problems with arousal and ejaculation. It's like the percussion part of the orchestra being out of sync with the rest of the players, causing a jarring and disjointed beat.

But here's the good news: hormonal imbalances are often treatable with lifestyle changes, medicines, or hormone replacement treatment. By addressing the underlying hormonal problems, people and couples can return balance to the symphony of sexual function, allowing for a more harmonious and satisfying experience of closeness.

Neurotransmitter Dysfunction:
Neurotransmitter dysfunction is similar to meeting roadblocks in the complex network of pathways within the brain, where each pathway is responsible for sending messages of pleasure and arousal. Imagine these paths as a complex system of roads, bustling with traffic carrying messages that control various bodily functions, including sexual reaction.

In this analogy, neurotransmitters are like the cars travelling along these roads, ferrying information between different parts of the brain. Among these neurotransmitters, serotonin and dopamine play crucial roles in influencing mood, pleasure, and excitement, all of which are important components of sexual function.

Now, picture a situation where these neurotransmitters meet dysfunction. It's like coming upon roadblocks along the highways of the brain, disrupting the smooth flow of traffic and causing delays in signal delivery. This disruption can appear as difficulties in getting and keeping arousal, as well as problems with controlling ejaculation.

For example, serotonin, often referred to as the "feel-good" neurotransmitter, is involved in managing mood and feeling. When serotonin levels are imbalanced, it can lead to mental disorders such as sadness and anxiety, which are known to be linked with sexual dysfunction, including premature ejaculation.

Similarly, dopamine, known as the "reward" neurotransmitter, plays a role in feeling pleasure and drive. Dysregulation of dopamine levels can impact the brain's response to sexual stimuli, possibly leading to problems in controlling ejaculation timing.

In essence, neurotransmitter failure can be likened to a disruption in the neural processes that control sexual function, leading to premature ejaculation. However, with proper evaluation and treatment, such as medicine or psychotherapy aimed at restoring neurotransmitter balance, people suffering this problem can often find relief and recover control over their sexual experiences.

3. Behavioural Habit:

Overstimulation:
Overstimulation is similar to lighting a firecracker in the night sky – a dazzling burst of energy that fades too quickly. Picture yourself in a state of heightened arousal, where every touch, feeling, and thought strengthens like sparks flying from a firework. This rush of pleasure can overwhelm the senses, leading to a premature climax before either partner is ready.

Imagine being at a show where the music is loud, the lights are bright, and the energy is obvious. In this situation, it's easy to become overstimulated, with the senses bombarded by a flood of sensory information. Similarly, during sexual action, overstimulation can occur when feelings become too intense, too quickly.

For example, picture engaging in sexual action after a long time of abstinence or heightened expectation. The anticipation and build-up of excitement can create a heightened state of sensitivity, making it easier to become overstimulated and reach climax quickly.

Moreover, certain sexual actions or methods, such as vigorous thrusting or intense stimulation of the penis, can also add to overstimulation. It's like revving the engine of a car too hard, burning through fuel at a fast pace and hitting the finish line before you meant.

Masturbation Habits:
Masturbation habits are similar to the currents of a river, shaping the landscape of sexual reaction over time. Picture a river running easily, its currents carving out pathways and reshaping the land with each ebb and flow. Similarly, masturbation habits can influence the body's response to sexual excitement and affect the time of ejaculation.

Imagine a person engaged in frequent and fast masturbation, often reaching climax quickly and with minimal stimulation. Over time, this pattern of behaviour can train the body to respond similarly during partnered sexual action. It's like carving a deep groove in the riverbank, guiding the flow of water along a set path.

On the other hand, someone who practises thoughtful and varied masturbation methods, exploring different feelings and pacing themselves, may develop a more nuanced and controlled reaction to sexual stimulation. It's like letting the water meander and branch out, making a diverse and dynamic scenery.

Furthermore, the content and setting of masturbation can also affect ejaculatory control. For example, individuals who frequently masturbate to pornography or participate in fantasy-driven stimulation may find it more challenging to maintain control during partnered sex, where the feelings and interactions are different. It's like sailing unfamiliar seas, where the currents of fantasy may not match with the flow of real-life closeness.

4. Medical Conditions:

Prostate Issues:
Prostate issues are similar to a stone thrown into a calm pond, upsetting the peaceful surface and causing waves across the water. Picture a quiet pond, its surface mirroring the peaceful surroundings like a mirror. Now, imagine a stone breaking the surface tension, causing waves that disturb the calmness of the water. Similarly, prostate issues can upset the delicate balance of sexual function, leading to rapid ejaculation.

The prostate gland, a small organ located just below the bladder, plays a key part in male sexual function. It produces a fluid that mixes with sperm to form semen, adding to ejaculation during sexual action. However, when the prostate gland becomes swollen or inflamed due to conditions such as prostatitis or benign prostatic hyperplasia (BPH), it can interfere with the usual process of ejaculation.

Picture the prostate gland as a highly tuned instrument, its smooth working necessary for the orchestration of sexual pleasure. When prostate problems appear, it's like a discordant note breaking the balance of the music, leading to difficulties in controlling ejaculation time.

For example, an enlarged prostate can put pressure on the urethra, the tube that takes pee and semen out of the body. This pressure can conflict with the usual flow of semen during ejaculation, causing it to be expelled soon. It's like a dam stopping the flow of water in a river, redirecting the stream and causing sudden waves.

Moreover, prostate inflammation or infection can cause discomfort or pain in the pelvic area, making it difficult to relax and fully engage in sexual activity. This discomfort can add to heightened arousal and sensitivity, increasing the chance of premature ejaculation. It's like trying to enjoy a peaceful swim in a turbulent sea, the waves of pain and distraction threatening to overcome.

Thyroid Disorders:
Thyroid disorders are like a faulty thermostat in the body's chemical control system, affecting the delicate balance of sexual function. Picture a thermostat controlling the temperature of a room, its settings ensuring the comfort of its users. Now, imagine that thermostat failing, causing the temperature to vary wildly. Similarly, thyroid disorders can upset the body's hormonal balance, affecting different parts of sexual performance.

The thyroid gland, found in the neck, produces hormones that control metabolism, energy levels, and numerous other bodily processes. When the thyroid gland is underactive (hypothyroidism) or hyperactive (hyperthyroidism), it can lead to a range of symptoms, including changes in libido, erectile dysfunction, and problems with orgasm and ejaculation.

Think of the thyroid gland as the director of an orchestra, leading the harmonious interplay of hormones that arrange sexual performance. When thyroid function is impaired, it's like a wayward director taking the orchestra wrong, resulting in discordant sounds and a lack of rhythm.

For example, in hypothyroidism, where the thyroid gland is sluggish and makes insufficient hormones, people may experience reduced libido and energy levels, as well as problems with arousal and orgasm. It's like trying to ignite a fire with damp wood, the sparks of desire fighting to catch flame amidst the lethargy and tiredness.

Conversely, in hyperthyroidism, where the thyroid gland is overactive and produces extra hormones, people may experience heightened arousal, anxiety, and rapid heartbeat, all of which can contribute to difficulties with ejaculation control. It's like a race car engine revving at full throttle, the excitement and energy overwhelming the ability to keep control.

2. Effects of Premature Ejaculation on Mental and Physical Well-being of Men: Navigating the Impact

Imagine sailing on the seas of closeness, with the goal of pleasure in sight. However, the trip is cut short by the sudden storm of premature ejaculation, leaving both lovers feeling adrift and unsatisfied. Premature ejaculation can have significant effects on the mental and physical well-being of men, disrupting the balance of closeness and leaving a wake of emotional and physical anguish. By recognizing and addressing these effects with kindness and care, individuals and couples can handle the challenges of premature ejaculation with resilience and understanding, eventually paving the way towards greater happiness and fulfilment in both mind and body.

Let's explore the ripple effects of premature ejaculation on the mental and physical well-being of guys, navigating the turbulent seas with care and understanding.

1. Mental Well-being:

Imagine standing on the edge of a cliff, with the possibility of closeness stretching out before you like a huge ocean. However, before you can fully immerse yourself in the experience, you find yourself falling into the depths of anger and self-doubt due to premature ejaculation. Premature ejaculation can cast a shadow over the mental well-being of men, creating a scene of inner turmoil and self-doubt. By recognizing and addressing these effects with kindness and understanding, individuals can begin to handle the challenges of premature ejaculation with grit and hope, eventually reclaiming their sense of self-worth and intimacy.
Let's dive deeper into the emotional whirlpool that premature ejaculation can cause, exploring its impact on the mental well-being of guys with empathy and clarity.

Performance Anxiety:
Imagine standing under a spotlight on a stage, every movement watched by an unknown crowd. Premature ejaculation can increase the fear of performance anxiety, changing private moments into a stage where one's sexual skills are put to the test.

The fear of failing a partner or not meeting their standards can burden the mind, causing feelings of inadequacy and doubt. It's like balancing on a wire between desire and dread, with the constant fear of failure hanging overhead.

Additionally, recurring instances of premature ejaculation can increase negative beliefs about one's sexual ability, increasing performance anxiety and diminishing self-esteem. It's like being stuck in a loop of self-criticism, where each setback confirms the belief that you're not skilled enough.

Relationship Strain:
Envision a garden where trust and intimacy thrive like delicate flowers, nurtured by the warmth of love. Premature ejaculation can resemble weeds, suffocating closeness and leaving both partners feeling detached and disconnected.

Coping with premature ejaculation can strain a relationship, creating stress and anger. It's similar to navigating a minefield of feelings, where each misstep widens the gap between partners.

Furthermore, the failure to fully please a partner may evoke feelings of guilt and inadequacy, intensifying the emotional strain. It's like carrying a heavy load on your shoulders, the weight of failed expectations getting heavier with each passing day.

Self-esteem and Confidence:
Visualise standing in front of a mirror, but instead of seeing yourself clearly, you see a distorted image looking back at you. Premature ejaculation can warp one's self-perception, causing feelings of shame and embarrassment.

The failure to control ejaculation can chip away at confidence and self-esteem, impacting how one sees themselves both inside and outside the bedroom. It's akin to wearing a mask of fake confidence, hiding real feelings behind a facade of bravado.

Additionally, the stigma surrounding rapid ejaculation can create a sense of isolation and shame, hindering the ability to seek support and understanding from others. It's like having a secret load, unable to confide in loved ones for fear of being judged or ridiculed.

2. Physical Well-being:

Premature ejaculation not only breaks the physical part of sexual pleasure but also inflicts emotional anguish, affecting mental well-being and the quality of relationships. By acknowledging these effects with understanding and compassion, people can begin to handle the challenges of premature ejaculation with resilience and hope, eventually aiming for greater happiness and fulfilment in both mind and body.

Sexual Satisfaction:
Premature ejaculation not only impedes the physical aspect of sexual satisfaction but also weakens the mental connection and happiness gained from close meetings. By recognizing and addressing the effect of premature ejaculation on sexual pleasure, individuals and couples can work towards improving closeness and creating a more enjoyable and successful sexual relationship.

Imagine preparing to start on a trip towards pleasure, filled with excitement and expectation, only to find yourself stopped before reaching the goal. Premature ejaculation can break the smooth flow of sexual pleasure, leaving both partners wishing for a more satisfying experience.

Physical closeness works as a cornerstone of general well-being, promoting connection, pleasure, and tenderness between partners. However, premature ejaculation can act as a barrier, hindering the achievement of full pleasure. It's like trying to quench your thirst with a leaky tap – the water trickles out inconsistently, failing to satiate your desire for satisfaction.

Moreover, the recurrence of premature ejaculation can plant seeds of anger and resentment within the fertile ground of closeness. This can negatively impact the quality of the relationship, leading to feelings of dissatisfaction and sadness. It's akin to sitting down to taste a delightful meal, only to have the pleasure constantly disrupted, leaving you hungry for more and unhappy with the experience.

Emotional Distress:
Premature ejaculation not only impacts physical well-being but also releases a cascade of emotional distress, pushing individuals to navigate through waves of embarrassment,

shame, and isolation. By recognizing and addressing these emotional effects with kindness and understanding, individuals can begin to chart a course towards healing and resilience, reclaiming their sense of self-worth and finding comfort in the support of others.

Imagine standing on the shore of your emotions, feeling the ground beneath your feet shift as waves of anger and sadness crash against the strong walls of your emotional stability. Premature ejaculation can unleash a storm of emotional turmoil, stirring up feelings of embarrassment, shame, and inadequacy that threaten to erode the very roots of your self-esteem.

Emotional distress acts as a heavy cloud that hangs over the scenery of happiness and satisfaction, obscuring the warmth of joy with its dark shadows. It's like being caught in a whirlpool of negative emotions, where each turn pulls you deeper into a sea of sadness, making it difficult to find solid ground.

Moreover, the shame surrounding premature ejaculation can shroud individuals in invisibility, hiding their problems from the outside world and leaving them feeling separated and alone in their pain. It's like wearing a mask of false bravado, pretending everything is fine while quietly fighting inner turmoil and self-doubt. This sense of isolation can create hurdles to finding support and understanding, leaving people feeling stranded in their battles, adrift in a sea of shame and secrecy.

3. Dispelling Myths and Misconceptions about Premature Ejaculation: Unveiling the Truth

Imagine stepping into a room filled with shadows of misunderstanding and lies surrounding premature ejaculation. Let's put light on these misconceptions, dispelling the myths that cloud our understanding and stopping people from getting help and support.

1. Myth: Premature Ejaculation is Rare

Truth: Premature ejaculation is more common than you might think, affecting guys of all ages and backgrounds. Research suggests that it's one of the most common sexual problems experienced by men, with figures showing that up to one-third of men may experience premature ejaculation at some point in their lives. It's important to recognize that having premature ejaculation doesn't mean there's something wrong with you—it's a common problem that many men face.

2. Myth: Premature Ejaculation is Always Caused by Psychological Issues

Truth: While psychological factors such as worry and stress can add to premature ejaculation, they're not the only factors at play. Biological factors like hormonal changes, nerve problems, and even certain medical conditions can also play a role. Additionally, relationship problems and behavioural habits may lead to premature ejaculation. It's important to consider the complex nature of premature ejaculation and address both psychological and physical factors when finding answers.

3. Myth: Premature Ejaculation is Untreatable

Truth: Contrary to popular opinion, premature ejaculation is a highly treatable disease. There are various methods and treatments available, ranging from behavioural techniques and routines to medicine and therapy. With the right direction and support, many men can successfully manage and overcome premature ejaculation, recovering control over their sexual experiences and improving their overall well-being.

4. Myth: Premature Ejaculation Only Affects Men

Truth: While premature ejaculation is usually linked with men, it can also impact their partners and the quality of their personal relationships. Partners may feel upset, unfulfilled, or separated due to premature ejaculation, leading to pressure and stress within the relationship. It's crucial for both partners to understand and handle premature ejaculation together, promoting open conversation, understanding, and support.

5. Myth: Premature Ejaculation is a Sign of Weakness or Inadequacy

Truth: Premature ejaculation is a common sexual problem that doesn't reflect a person's manhood, power, or worth. It's important to question the misconception that having premature ejaculation makes someone weak or inadequate. Instead, it's a natural part of human sexuality that can be handled with compassion, understanding, and proper treatment.

6. Myth: Premature Ejaculation is Always a Chronic Condition

Truth: While some cases of premature ejaculation may continue over time, it's not always a chronic problem. Many people experience occasional cases of premature ejaculation due to situational factors such as stress, tiredness, or relationship problems. These episodes may resolve on their own or with easy treatments, such as relaxation methods or conversation with a partner. It's important to know that having rare premature ejaculation doesn't necessarily mean it will become a long-term problem.

7. Myth: Premature Ejaculation Only Occurs During Intercourse

Truth: While premature ejaculation typically happens during penetrative intercourse, it can also occur during other sexual activities, such as foreplay or masturbation. The focus on penetrative intercourse as the main measure of sexual success can add to feelings of inadequacy and pressure, further exacerbating premature ejaculation. It's important to broaden our knowledge of sexual experiences and recognize that pleasure and closeness can take many forms beyond intercourse.

8. Myth: Premature Ejaculation is a Normal Part of Aging

Truth: While it's true that sexual function may change with age, premature ejaculation is not a necessary result of ageing. While some older men may experience changes in sexual function, including delayed ejaculation, it's not considered a normal part of the ageing process. Premature ejaculation can occur at any age and may be affected by various factors, including health problems, medicines, and lifestyle factors. It's important to handle premature ejaculation regardless of age and seek suitable help if needed.

9. Myth: Premature Ejaculation is solely the Man's Responsibility

Truth: While premature ejaculation may primarily affect men, handling it is a shared duty within a relationship. Partners can play a crucial part in giving support, understanding, and motivation during the treatment process. Open conversation, empathy, and shared understanding can help improve the bond between partners and create a supportive atmosphere for handling premature ejaculation together.

10. Myth: Premature Ejaculation is a Taboo Topic

Truth: Despite the shame surrounding premature ejaculation, talking it freely and getting help is important for handling the problem successfully. Keeping premature ejaculation secret or avoiding talks about it can perpetuate feelings of shame and isolation. By breaking the silence and getting help from healthcare professionals, partners, or support groups, people can find the guidance and resources needed to manage premature ejaculation and improve their sexual well-being.

11. Myth: Premature Ejaculation is Always a Sign of Sexual Dysfunction

Truth: While premature ejaculation is considered a type of sexual dysfunction, having occasional episodes does not necessarily indicate an ongoing or serious problem. It's important to differentiate between occasional premature ejaculation, which may be due to situational factors or brief problems, and chronic premature ejaculation, which may require more focused action. Understanding the range of premature ejaculation can help people and couples handle their experiences more successfully and seek suitable support when needed.

12. Myth: Premature Ejaculation Can Be Cured Overnight

Truth: Treating premature ejaculation often takes patience, determination, and a multifaceted approach. While some people may experience changes with simple techniques or treatments, such as behavioural strategies or communication exercises, addressing premature ejaculation effectively may take time and trial. It's essential to approach treatment with realistic goals and a willingness to explore different methods to find what works best for each individual's unique needs and circumstances.

13. Myth: Premature Ejaculation Only Affects Men with High Libido

Truth: Premature ejaculation can affect people across the range of libido levels, from those with high sexual desire to those with lower levels of interest. While factors such as arousal strength and sexual regularity may affect the experience of premature ejaculation, it can occur in people with different levels of libido and sexual activity.

Understanding that premature ejaculation can affect anyone, regardless of their libido level, can help reduce shame and support open talks about the problem.

14. Myth: Premature Ejaculation is Always a Sign of Relationship Problems

Truth: While relationship problems can add to premature ejaculation for some people, it's not always the main cause. Premature ejaculation can stem from a variety of factors, including biological, psychological, and situational factors, regardless of the health of the relationship. While addressing relationship issues can be helpful for general sexual health and satisfaction, it's important to consider and address other possible causes adding to premature ejaculation to effectively control the condition.

15. Myth: Premature Ejaculation Treatment Is One-Size-Fits-All

Truth: Effective treatment for premature ejaculation varies based on individual needs, tastes, and underlying factors adding to the condition. What works for one person may not work for another, and it may take some trial and error to find the most effective method.

Treatment choices range from behavioural methods and exercises to medicines, therapy, and lifestyle changes. Tailoring treatment to each individual's unique circumstances is important for optimising results and improving general sexual well-being.

16. Myth: Premature Ejaculation Is Always a Result of Poor Sexual Technique

Truth: While sexual methods can play a role in premature ejaculation for some people, it's not always the main reason. Premature ejaculation can be affected by a wide range of factors, including biological, psychological, and relationship aspects. Blaming poor sexual skill skips the complexity of premature ejaculation and may lead to feelings of inadequacy and anger. It's important to approach premature ejaculation with a thorough understanding and study various factors that may contribute to its occurrence.

17. Myth: Premature Ejaculation Is Not a Serious Concern

Truth: Premature ejaculation can have significant effects on an individual's quality of life, relationships, and general well-being. Beyond the physical part, it can lead to mental discomfort, low self-esteem, and problems in interpersonal relationships. Ignoring or dismissing premature ejaculation as a small problem can perpetuate feelings of shame and hinder people from getting help and support. Recognizing the importance of addressing premature ejaculation and its possible effects is crucial for promoting sexual health and general happiness.

18. Myth: Premature Ejaculation Only Affects Younger Men

Truth: While premature ejaculation is often linked with younger guys, it can occur at any age. While incidence may be higher among younger people, premature ejaculation can affect men of all ages, including older adults. Biological, social, and lifestyle factors can lead to premature ejaculation regardless of age. Understanding that premature ejaculation is not limited to younger men can help spread understanding and urge people of all ages to seek support and treatment if needed.

19. Myth: Premature Ejaculation Is Just a Phase
That Will Resolve Itself

Truth: While some cases of rapid ejaculation may
settle on their own, it's not always the case for
everyone. Persistent premature ejaculation may
require intervention and treatment to address
underlying causes adding to the condition.
Waiting for premature ejaculation to fix itself
without taking deliberate steps to address it may
lengthen distress and hinder overall sexual
well-being. Seeking help and support can enable
people to take control of their sexual health and
improve their quality of life.

20. Myth: Premature Ejaculation Is Always
Caused by Excessive Sexual Activity

Truth: While excessive sexual activity may lead
to premature ejaculation for some people, it's not
the main cause of the condition. Premature
ejaculation can be affected by a variety of
factors, including biological, social, and relational
features. Blaming premature ejaculation solely
on sexual activity ignores the complexity of the
problem and may lead to mistakes and
misconceptions. It's important to consider a
broad approach to premature ejaculation and
study various factors adding to its occurrence.

By dispelling these myths and misconceptions, we can create a more helpful and understanding atmosphere for people having premature ejaculation. It's time to shine a light on the truth and empower people to seek the help and support they need to overcome premature ejaculation and improve their sexual well-being.

Chapter Two:

Lifestyle Changes for Overcoming Premature Ejaculation

Embarking on a trip toward enhanced sexual performance and happiness requires more than just a fleeting glance at quick fixes. It includes a holistic method that embraces living changes aimed at nurturing both body and mind. In this study, we dive into the world of diet modifications, exercise routines, and stress management methods, each giving a key to unlocking the door to prolonged pleasure and intimacy. Join us as we navigate the seas of potential, charting a path toward a more fulfilling and satisfying sexual experience. In our drive to beat premature ejaculation, we turn to lifestyle changes as potent tools in our arsenal. These changes offer not only instant benefits but also long-term solutions for reclaiming power and prolonging pleasure in the bedroom.

1. Diet Modifications: Foods That Can Help Delay Ejaculation
A careful approach to nutrition can offer significant benefits in controlling premature ejaculation. Certain foods and dietary choices

have been linked to better sexual energy and control. By adding nutrient-rich foods into our diet and avoiding causes that may worsen premature ejaculation, we can optimise our body's physiological reactions and extend the length of intimate encounters. From the aphrodisiac properties of certain fruits to the stamina-boosting effects of protein-rich foods, our dietary choices can play a pivotal role in improving sexual performance and happiness.

2. Exercise and Physical Activity: Benefits for Sexual Stamina
Regular exercise not only adds to general physical fitness but also has deep effects on sexual health and energy. Engaging in a regular exercise routine can improve cardiovascular health, boost circulation, and increase endurance—all of which are crucial components of sexual function. By incorporating exercises that target pelvic floor muscles and promote relaxation, people can improve their ability to control ejaculation and lengthen the time of sexual activity. From yoga poses that promote awareness to cardio workouts that improve stamina, exercise offers a varied approach to beating premature ejaculation and improving sexual pleasure.

3. Stress Management Techniques: Relaxation Methods to Reduce Performance Anxiety
Stress and worry are common causes behind premature ejaculation, often worsening the condition and hindering sexual performance. Learning effective stress management techniques can be helpful in easing performance anxiety and boosting relaxation during intimate meetings. From deep breathing exercises and meditation practices to mindfulness techniques and progressive muscle relaxation, people can develop a sense of calm and presence that empowers them to handle sexual situations with confidence and ease. By addressing the root causes of stress and anxiety, we can create a helpful environment for overcoming premature ejaculation and encouraging closeness and connection with our partners.

In our search for lasting pleasure and happiness, these lifestyle changes serve as pillars of support, leading us toward a more satisfying and enriching sexual experience. By adopting diet modifications, exercise routines, and stress management techniques, we empower ourselves to take control of our sexual health and well-being, paving the way for greater intimacy, pleasure, and happiness in the bedroom.

1. Diet Modifications: Foods That Can Help Delay Ejaculation

Embarking on a journey toward better physical success starts on our plates. A careful approach to eating isn't just about feeding our bodies—it's about nourishing our sexual health too. Let's explore how certain foods can become our friends in managing premature ejaculation and prolonging the pleasure of intimate times.

Aphrodisiac Fruits: Fueling Passion and Prolonging Pleasure

Picture yourself revelling in nature's sweet pleasures, each bite awakening your senses and stirring the flames of desire. Aphrodisiac fruits hold the promise of not only tantalising your taste buds but also sparking your desire, offering a delicious route to enhanced sexual energy and control. Let's discover these tantalising gems and their potential to lengthen the pleasure of intimate moments:

1. Bananas:
Bananas are not just a handy snack; they are also rich in nutrients that support sexual health. Loaded with potassium, an essential mineral for muscle function, bananas help control blood pressure and promote healthy circulation—an

important factor in getting and keeping erections. Additionally, the bromelain enzyme found in bananas may help boost libido and sexual energy, making them a natural choice for those looking to delay ejaculation.

2. Avocados:
Creamy, delicious avocados are more than just a trendy toast topper—they are a powerhouse of nutrients known to improve sexual energy. Rich in vitamin E, bananas support cardiovascular health and improve blood flow throughout the body, including to the groin area. This better circulation can contribute to stronger and longer-lasting erections, helping to delay ejaculation and increase sexual pleasure.

3. Figs:
Bursting with sweetness and sensuality, figs have long been adored for their aphrodisiac qualities. These delicious fruits are packed with important nutrients like potassium, magnesium, and antioxidants, which support general sexual health. Figs are particularly rich in arginine, an amino acid that plays a key role in the production of nitric oxide—a substance that relaxes blood vessels and improves blood flow to the penis. By promoting healthy circulation, figs can help improve erectile function and delay ejaculation,

allowing for more pleasurable and longer sexual experiences.

4. Watermelon:
Refreshing and hydrating, watermelon is not only a summer favourite but also a natural enhancer of sexual function. This juicy fruit is rich in citrulline, an amino acid that the body turns into arginine—a precursor to nitric oxide. Increased amounts of nitric oxide can improve blood flow to the genitals, resulting in bigger and longer-lasting erections. By adding watermelon into your diet, you can support healthy erectile function and increase the length of sexual intercourse.

5. Pomegranates:
With their vibrant ruby-red seeds and tangy-sweet taste, pomegranates are a sign of fertility and desire. These antioxidant-rich fruits contain compounds that promote cardiovascular health and increase blood flow, making them useful partners in the fight for sexual vitality. Pomegranate juice has been shown to improve erectile function and delay ejaculation, offering a natural option for those looking to lengthen their sexual pleasure.

6. Mangoes:
Sweet, juicy mangoes are not only a tropical
treat but also a source of energy and sensuality.
Rich in vitamin C and vitamin E, mangoes
promote healthy blood circulation and support
cardiovascular health—essential factors for good
sexual function. Additionally, mangoes contain
beta-carotene, a precursor to vitamin A, which is
known to boost libido and improve sexual
pleasure.

7. Strawberries:
Plump, ripe strawberries are not just a sign of
romance but also a powerful aphrodisiac. These
delicious berries are packed with antioxidants like
vitamin C and flavonoids, which help improve
blood flow and boost heart health. Additionally,
strawberries are rich in folate, a vitamin that
supports the production of sex hormones and
improves sexual pleasure. Enjoying a bowl of
strawberries with your partner can excite the
senses and set the mood for a passionate
meeting.

8. Grapes:
Whether eaten fresh or as a glass of wine,
grapes have long been linked with love and
fertility. Grapes contain resveratrol, a strong
antioxidant that supports cardiovascular health

and improves blood flow. By promoting healthy
circulation, grapes can improve erectile
performance and prolong sexual endurance.
Additionally, the act of feeding each other grapes
can be a sensual and personal experience,
increasing arousal and strengthening the
connection between lovers.

9. Pineapples:
Tangy and tropical, pineapples are not only a
delicious treat but also a sign of welcome and
romance. These unusual fruits are rich in
bromelain, an enzyme that has been shown to
improve blood flow and lower inflammation. By
supporting healthy circulation, pineapples can
improve erectile function and delay ejaculation,
leading to more pleasurable and longer sexual
experiences. Additionally, the sweet and
refreshing flavour of pineapples can stir the taste
buds and awaken the senses, adding an extra
layer of excitement to intimate meetings.

10. Cherries:
 With their ruby-red hue and sweet-tart taste,
cherries are a tempting indulgence that can
spark love and desire. These tiny fruits are rich
in antioxidants like anthocyanins, which help
improve blood flow and protect against oxidative
stress. By promoting healthy circulation, cherries

can improve erectile function and increase sexual energy. Additionally, the act of sharing cherries with your partner can be a playful and personal move, promoting intimacy and connection in the bedroom.

By enjoying these aphrodisiac foods as part of a balanced diet, you can nourish your body with important nutrients and support healthy sexual function. From potassium-rich bananas to antioxidant-packed pomegranates, nature's bounty offers a delicious array of options for lengthening the pleasure of intimate moments and fueling the flames of passion.

Protein-Packed Powerhouses: Strengthening Your Sexual Stamina

Imagine indulging in a hearty meal that not only feeds your body but also improves your sexual prowess. Protein-rich foods like chicken, fish, and tofu offer more than just satiety—they provide the necessary building blocks for improving the muscles involved in ejaculation control. Let's explore how adding these protein-packed powerhouses into our diet can lead to longer-lasting and more enjoyable sexual encounters:

1. Chicken:
Lean and flexible, chicken is a staple energy source that can support your sexual health and performance. Packed with important amino acids like L-arginine and L-carnitine, chicken helps support healthy blood flow and improve erectile performance. Additionally, the high protein content in chicken supports muscle growth and repair, including the pelvic floor muscles responsible for controlling ejaculation. By having grilled chicken breast or roasted chicken thighs as part of your regular meals, you can fortify your body with the nutrients it needs to delay ejaculation and increase sexual pleasure.

2. Fish:
From salmon to tuna to mackerel, fatty fish are rich in omega-3 fatty acids—a nutrient important for cardiovascular health and sexual function. Omega-3s help improve blood circulation and artery dilation, leading to improved erectile performance and longer sexual energy. Moreover, fish is a high-quality protein source that offers the amino acids necessary for muscle repair and growth. By adding fatty fish into your diet two to three times per week, you can support optimal sexual health and function while having delicious and nutritious meals.

3. Tofu:

For those following a plant-based diet or trying to lower their meat usage, tofu offers a versatile and protein-rich alternative. Made from soybeans, tofu is a complete protein source that offers all the necessary amino acids your body needs for muscle health and repair. Additionally, tofu is low in saturated fat and cholesterol, making it a heart-healthy choice that supports general cardiovascular performance. By adding tofu into stir-fries, salads, or smoothies, you can fuel your body with plant-based protein and strengthen the muscles involved in ejaculation control, leading to better sexual energy and pleasure.

4. Eggs:

Versatile and nutrient-rich, eggs are a breakfast staple that can also support your sexual health. Egg whites are particularly high in protein, giving the amino acids necessary for muscle repair and growth. Additionally, eggs are rich in vitamins and minerals like vitamin D and zinc, which play key roles in testosterone production and general sexual function. Whether eaten scrambled, poached, or boiled, adding eggs into your diet can help strengthen your pelvic floor muscles and delay ejaculation.

5. Lean Beef:
Beef is a rich source of protein and important nutrients like iron and zinc, which are crucial for sexual health and performance. Lean cuts of beef, such as sirloin or tenderloin, provide high-quality protein with less saturated fat, making them a heart-healthy choice for boosting sexual energy. Additionally, the amino acid presence in beef helps support muscle growth and repair, including the muscles involved in ejaculation control. Enjoying a grilled steak or beef stir-fry can not only please your taste buds but also fuel your sexual ability.

6. Greek Yoghourt:
Creamy and luxurious, Greek yoghurt is not only a delicious snack but also a powerful source of protein and probiotics. Greek yoghurt includes twice the protein of regular yoghurt, making it an excellent choice for supporting muscle growth and repair. Additionally, the probiotics in Greek yoghurt promote digestive health and may indirectly help to better sexual function by supporting general well-being. Whether eaten plain or topped with fruit and nuts, Greek yoghurt can be a satisfying and nutritious addition to your diet for improving sexual stamina.

7. Quinoa:
As a full protein source, quinoa offers all nine
necessary amino acids, making it an ideal choice
for vegetarians and vegans looking to boost their
protein intake. Quinoa is also rich in fibre,
vitamins, and minerals, including magnesium and
iron, which support general health and energy.
By adding quinoa into your meals, such as
salads, soups, or stir-fries, you can fuel your
body with the nutrients it needs to strengthen
your pelvic floor muscles and prevent
ejaculation.

8. Cottage Cheese:
Creamy and filling, cottage cheese is a dairy
product that's rich in protein and low in fat. It
offers a slow-release source of protein, which can
help keep you feeling full and satisfied for longer
times. Additionally, cottage cheese is a good
source of calcium and phosphorus, important
minerals that support bone health and muscle
function. Enjoy cottage cheese as a snack or
work it into your meals to support muscle growth
and delay ejaculation.

Incorporating protein-packed powerhouses into
your diet is not just about filling your
hunger—it's about improving your sexual health

and performance. By nourishing your body with lean proteins and important nutrients, you can strengthen your pelvic floor muscles, improve blood flow, and delay ejaculation, leading to longer-lasting and more satisfying sexual encounters.

Whether you prefer eggs for breakfast, beef for dinner, or Greek yoghurt for a snack, there are plenty of delicious and nutritious choices to fuel your sexual prowess and improve your pleasure in the bedroom.
Enjoy those grilled chicken breasts, indulge in a seafood feast, or whip up a tofu stir-fry—your sexual power awaits!

Omega-3-Rich Delights: Fueling Your Sexual Vitality

Imagine indulging in a culinary treat that not only tantalises your taste buds but also feeds your body from within. Omega-3-rich foods like fatty fish, nuts, and seeds offer a delectable route to better sexual health and function. Let's explore these nutritional powerhouses and their potential to improve your sexual energy and satisfaction:

1. Salmon:
Picture enjoying a perfectly grilled salmon fillet, its tender meat melting in your mouth with each delicious bite. Salmon is not only a delicious seafood treat but also a rich source of omega-3 fatty acids, especially EPA and DHA. These important fatty acids play a key part in cardiovascular health by reducing inflammation, lowering blood pressure, and improving blood vessel function. By promoting healthy circulation, salmon helps ensure proper blood flow to the genitals, leading to bigger and longer-lasting erections. Incorporating salmon into your diet two to three times a week can support good sexual function and pleasure.

2. Flaxseeds:
Envision spreading golden flaxseed oil over your salad or adding ground flaxseeds to your morning smoothie—simple yet powerful ways to boost your omega-3 diet. Flaxseeds are rich in alpha-linolenic acid (ALA), a plant-based omega-3 fatty acid that offers numerous health benefits, including better circulatory function. ALA helps lower inflammation and support blood vessel health, leading to improved blood flow throughout the body, including to the penis. By adding flaxseeds or flaxseed oil into your daily

diet, you can support good erectile function and improve your sexual stamina over time.

3. Walnuts:
Imagine cracking open a fresh walnut and revelling in its rich, buttery flavour—a sensory experience that not only fills your taste buds but also feeds your body with important nutrients. Walnuts are a rich source of omega-3 fatty acids, especially ALA, which has been linked to better cardiovascular health and sexual function. Additionally, walnuts contain arginine, an amino acid that promotes nitric oxide production—a substance that softens blood vessels and improves blood flow. By having a handful of walnuts as a snack or incorporating them into your meals, you can support healthy blood circulation and enhance your sexual energy.

4. Chia Seeds:
Picture sprinkling chia seeds over your morning breakfast or mixing them into a refreshing smoothie—a simple yet effective way to boost your omega-3 intake. Chia seeds are rich in ALA, fibre, and antioxidants, making them a nutritional powerhouse for supporting general health and energy. The omega-3 fatty acids in chia seeds help lower inflammation, support heart health, and improve blood flow, all of which

are important for optimal sexual function. By adding chia seeds into your diet regularly, you can enhance your cardiovascular health and promote greater sexual energy and pleasure.

5. Sardines:
Imagine enjoying the robust flavour of grilled sardines, their soft meat filled with omega-3 goodness. Sardines are a small, oily fish packed with EPA and DHA omega-3 fatty acids, which are important for cardiovascular health and sexual function. These fatty acids help reduce inflammation, lower blood pressure, and improve blood vessel activity, leading to improved blood flow and stronger erections. Incorporating sardines into your diet can provide a delicious and healthy boost to your sexual energy.

6. Hemp Seeds:
Picture sprinkling nutty-tasting hemp seeds over your morning yoghurt or salad—a simple yet powerful way to increase your omega-3 diet. Hemp seeds are rich in ALA omega-3 fatty acids, as well as protein, fibre, and important vitamins and minerals. The combination of nutrients in hemp seeds improves cardiovascular health, reduces inflammation, and enhances blood flow, all of which are helpful for sexual performance. Adding hemp seeds to your daily diet can help to

improve sexual stamina and happiness over time.

7. Mackerel:

Envision enjoying a delicious grilled mackerel piece, its rich flavour and flaky texture a testament to its omega-3 content. Mackerel is a fatty fish that offers a large dose of EPA and DHA omega-3 fatty acids, along with protein and other important nutrients. These fatty acids support cardiovascular health, lower inflammation, and improve blood vessel function, leading to improved blood flow and erectile performance. Incorporating mackerel into your diet can help promote ideal sexual function and pleasure.

8. Algal Oil:

Imagine spreading algae oil over your salad or using it as a cooking oil—a plant-based alternative to fish oil that offers the same omega-3 benefits. Algal oil is produced from algae, a rich source of DHA omega-3 fatty acids, which are important for brain health, heart health, and sexual function. Algal oil provides a vegan-friendly choice for increasing your omega-3 diet, improving cardiovascular health, and enhancing sexual vitality without the need for fish-based sources.

By adding these omega-3-rich foods into your diet, you can nourish your body with important nutrients and support your sexual health and performance. Whether you're enjoying grilled sardines, sprinkling hemp seeds over your meals, succulent salmon fillet, sprinkling flaxseeds over your salad, munching on walnuts as a snack, or drizzling algal oil over your dishes, these delicious and nutritious foods offer a tasty way to boost your omega-3 intake and enhance your sexual vitality.

Spice Up Your Life: Igniting Passion with Flavor

Imagine a culinary adventure where every bite ignites your feelings and fuels your desire for closeness. Spice up your meals with ingredients like garlic, chilli peppers, and ginger—flavours that not only excite your taste buds but also awaken your libido. Let's explore how these spicy treats can add a bit of excitement to your love life:

1. Garlic:
Picture the aromatic aroma of garlic sizzling in a pan, filling your foods with its rich and savoury flavour. Beyond its culinary allure, garlic is believed to have aphrodisiac qualities that can

improve sexual desire and ability. Garlic contains allicin, a substance that promotes blood flow and cardiovascular health, leading to better circulation and heightened arousal. By adding garlic into your meals, you can spice up your love life while getting the health benefits of this versatile vegetable.

2. Chili Peppers:
Envision sinking your teeth into a hot chilli pepper, its heat sparking a passionate spark within you. Chilli peppers contain capsaicin, a compound that stimulates nerve ends and increases heart rate, causing a feeling of energy and arousal. The spicy kick of chilli peppers can boost circulation and trigger the release of endorphins, improving pleasure and strengthening feelings during intimate moments. Whether eaten raw, cooked, or as a spicy sauce, chilli peppers can add a hot flair to your love life.

3. Ginger:
Imagine sipping on a warm cup of ginger tea, its spicy warmth moving through your body and waking your senses. Ginger is prized for its aphrodisiac qualities and has been used for ages to enhance sexual desire and performance. This delicious root includes gingerol, a compound that improves blood flow and circulation, leading to

heightened awareness and excitement. Adding
ginger to your meals or having it in tea can spice
up your love life while promoting general health
and well-being.

4. Saffron:
Picture the vivid hues of saffron infusing your
meals with a touch of luxury and sensuality.
Saffron is one of the world's most expensive
herbs and has been prized for its aphrodisiac
powers since ancient times. This exotic spice
contains compounds that trigger serotonin
release and improve mood, leading to greater
sexual desire and pleasure. Whether used in
savoury recipes or sweet treats, saffron adds a
bit of romance and indulgence to your culinary
creations, making every meal a feast for the
senses.

5. Cinnamon:
Picture the warm and welcoming aroma of
cinnamon wafting through your kitchen, evoking
memories of cosy nights and sweet indulgence.
Beyond its lovely taste, cinnamon is believed to
have aphrodisiac qualities that can improve
sexual desire and pleasure. This aromatic spice
includes chemicals that promote blood flow and
circulation, leading to greater sensitivity and
arousal. Whether put on your morning oatmeal

or added to a romantic treat, cinnamon can add a bit of sweetness and sexiness to your culinary creations.

6. Cardamom:
Imagine the exotic smell of cardamom filling the air, transporting you to faraway places and old customs. Cardamom is prized for its aromatic taste and medicinal qualities, including its ability to improve sexual desire and performance. This fragrant spice contains chemicals that increase blood flow and improve circulation, leading to heightened awareness and arousal. Whether used in savoury recipes or sweet treats, cardamom adds a touch of elegance and intrigue to your cooking repertoire, making every meal a sensual experience.

7. Vanilla:
Envision the rich and creamy aroma of vanilla bean dancing in your favourite dessert, its intoxicating scent captivating your senses. Vanilla is more than just a flavouring—it's a sign of romance and pleasure, with aphrodisiac properties that have been admired for centuries. This sweet and subtle spice contains compounds that boost mood and promote relaxation, creating a feeling of closeness and connection. Whether infused in a delicious custard or added

to a luxurious bath, vanilla can improve your sensual experiences and spark love in the bedroom.

8. Nutmeg:
Picture the warm and earthy flavour of nutmeg gracing your holiday desserts, its mild spice adding depth and complexity to your culinary creations. Nutmeg is known for its aromatic fragrance and aphrodisiac qualities, thought to improve sexual desire and ability. This flexible spice contains chemicals that boost blood flow and increase sensitivity, leading to heightened arousal and pleasure. Whether grated over a creamy pasta dish or sprinkled on a frothy latte, nutmeg can add a bit of warmth and sensuality to your romantic times.

Incorporating these aromatic spices and herbs into your meals can add a layer of excitement and sexiness to your love life.

Whether you're indulging in the warm embrace of cinnamon, the exotic allure of cardamom, or the sweet indulgence of vanilla, whether you're cooking up a garlic-infused masterpiece, indulging in the fiery heat of chilli peppers, or savouring the exotic allure of saffron, these flavorful ingredients can ignite passion and awaken your senses, making every encounter a feast for the soul.

Incorporating these foods into our diet isn't just about filling our hunger—it's about supporting our sexual health and improving our pleasure in the bedroom. By accepting a diet rich in aphrodisiac fruits, protein-packed powerhouses, omega-3-rich treats, and spices that spice up our life, we can optimise our body's physiological reactions and extend the length of personal encounters, leading to greater happiness and fulfilment for both partners.

2. Exercise and Physical Activity: Building Sexual Stamina

Imagine starting on a journey toward better sexual health and satisfaction—one that starts with a simple step: regular exercise. It's not just about getting in shape; it's about releasing your full ability in the bedroom. Incorporating these movements into your routine, you're not just improving your physical fitness; you're also enhancing your sexual health and happiness. From boosting blood flow to strengthening pelvic muscles, exercise offers a complete answer to premature ejaculation. So lace up those sneakers, roll out your yoga mat, and get ready to take your sexual energy to new heights.

Here's how exercise can change your sexual energy and help you beat premature ejaculation:

1. Cardiovascular Workouts: Think of cardio workouts like jogging, swimming, or cycling as your ticket to better sexual function. These activities get your heart moving and improve blood circulation throughout your body, including to your groin area. With better blood flow comes bigger and longer-lasting erections, allowing you to stay in the game for longer and enjoy more satisfying sexual encounters.

2. Strength Training: Imagine yourself lifting weights or doing basic workouts like push-ups and squats. Strength training not only grows muscle but also boosts general endurance, crucial for maintaining sexual activity. By targeting key muscle groups, including those in your pelvic floor, you can gain better control over your ejaculation and extend your sexual energy.

3. Yoga and Relaxation Techniques: Envision finding your inner calm and balance through yoga and mindfulness techniques. Yoga poses and relaxation methods not only lower stress but

also improve your pelvic floor muscles. With greater control over these muscles, you can delay ejaculation and increase sexual pleasure. Plus, the awareness gained from these activities helps you stay present and fully engaged during intimate times.

4. Kegel Exercises: Picture yourself quietly squeezing and relaxing your pelvic floor muscles throughout the day. These Kegel movements are like a hidden weapon against premature ejaculation, as they strengthen the muscles responsible for controlling ejaculation. With regular practice, you can improve your ability to hold back and extend your sexual performance.

5. Interval Training: Imagine switching between bursts of high-intensity exercise and times of rest or lower intensity. Interval training not only burns calories and improves cardiovascular health but also increases endurance and energy. By pushing your body with short bursts of intense activity followed by rest times, you can build strength and energy in the bedroom.

6. Core Strengthening Exercises: Picture yourself engaged in movements that target your core muscles, including planks, Russian twists, and leg raises. A strong core not only improves

balance and stability but also enhances total physical performance, including sexual energy. By strengthening your core muscles, you can keep better control and stability during intimate moments, leading to more prolonged and satisfying sexual meetings.

7. Pelvic Floor Exercises for Men: Envision performing specific exercises meant to strengthen the muscles of the pelvic floor, such as pelvic floor contractions (also known as Kegels) and reverse Kegels. These exercises help improve muscle tone and control in the pelvic area, allowing you to better manage your ejaculation and delay climax during sexual activity. By adding pelvic floor exercises into your routine, you can improve your sexual stamina and ability over time.

8. Tai Chi and Qi Gong: Imagine moving through gentle, fluid moves that promote relaxing, balance, and energy flow throughout your body. Tai Chi and Qi Gong are old Chinese martial arts methods that focus on mindfulness, breath control, and gentle movements. These techniques not only reduce stress and worry but also improve circulation and energy levels, leading to improved sexual vitality and stamina. By adding Tai Chi or Qi Gong into your routine,

you can develop a sense of inner harmony and physical well-being that translates into better sexual performance.

9. Squats: Imagine lowering your body into a seated position, then rising back up again, working your glutes, hamstrings, and quads. Squats are a compound exercise that not only builds your lower body but also uses your core muscles and improves balance. By adding squats into your workout routine, you can build general strength and endurance, enhancing your ability to continue sexual activity for longer durations.

10. Deadlifts: Picture yourself moving a weighted barbell from the ground to a standing stance, working your full posterior chain, including your glutes, hamstrings, and lower back. Deadlifts are a useful strength practice that not only builds muscle mass but also improves grip strength and stability. By performing deadlifts regularly, you can build greater general strength and resilience, adding to better sexual stamina and performance.

11. Cycling: Envision yourself pedalling through beautiful scenery, feeling the wind against your face and the rhythm of the ride pushing you forward. Cycling is an excellent cardiovascular

exercise that not only burns calories but also builds your lower body muscles and improves stamina. By adding riding into your exercise routine, you can improve your cardiovascular health, boost circulation, and build leg strength, all of which are beneficial for sexual energy.

12. Swimming: Picture yourself gliding through the water with easy ease, feeling the resistance of the water against your muscles as you push yourself forward. Swimming is a low-impact, full-body workout that not only improves cardiovascular health but also grows muscular strength and stamina. By swimming daily, you can increase lung capacity, improve circulation, and boost general physical fitness, leading to better sexual stamina and performance.
Of course! Here are a few more examples of workouts that can help improve sexual energy and address premature ejaculation:

13. Box Jumps: Imagine explosively jumping onto a higher platform, using the power of your legs to launch yourself upward. Box jumps are plyometric workouts that not only build lower body strength but also improve explosive power and speed. By adding box jumps into your workout routine, you can enhance your general

athleticism and stamina, leading to better performance in the bedroom.

14. Rowing: Picture yourself flowing through the water, pulling the oars with rhythmic accuracy and feeling the burn in your upper body and core. Rowing is a full-body workout that not only improves physical health but also builds muscles in the arms, shoulders, back, and core. By incorporating rowing into your exercise routine, you can improve endurance, increase muscle tone, and enhance general physical fitness, leading to better sexual stamina and performance.

15. Jump Rope: Envision the rhythmic sound of the jump rope hitting the ground as you jump with speed and precision, feeling your heart rate rise with each turn. Jump rope is a high-intensity cardiovascular workout that not only burns calories but also improves coordination, balance, and stamina. By adding jump rope into your practice, you can enhance cardiovascular health, increase stamina, and improve general physical conditioning, all of which contribute to better sexual performance.

16. Burpees: Picture yourself going from a standing position to a plank, then performing a push-up before explosively jumping back up to standing, continuing the movement with fluidity and control. Burpees are a full-body workout that not only builds strength and endurance but also raises heart rate and burns calories. By adding burpees into your workout routine, you can improve cardiovascular health, increase muscular endurance, and boost general physical fitness, leading to better sexual energy and performance.

By including a range of workouts in your routine, you can target different muscle groups, improve cardiovascular health, and enhance general physical fitness, eventually leading to better sexual energy and performance. Whether you're engaging in interval training, building your core, practising pelvic floor exercises, or exploring the gentle moves of Tai Chi and Qi Gong, each exercise offers unique benefits that contribute to your sexual health and happiness.

3. Stress Management Techniques: Finding Calm Amidst the Storm

Imagine being able to step into times of intimacy with confidence and ease, free from the grip of fear and worry. Learning effective stress management methods can unlock the door to a more fulfilling and happy sex life, allowing you to overcome premature ejaculation and welcome closeness with open arms. Let's explore some relaxing methods and mindfulness practices that can help you reduce performance anxiety and develop a sense of calmness and presence in the bedroom:

1. Deep Breathing Exercises: Picture yourself taking slow, deep breaths, breathing through your nose and exhaling through your mouth, feeling the stress melt away with each breath. Deep breathing techniques are a powerful tool for calming the nervous system and reducing worry and anxiety. By focusing on your breath and taking slow, deliberate breaths, you can activate the body's relaxation response, promoting a sense of calmness and centeredness that can take you through private moments with ease.

2. Meditation Practices: Envision carving out a few moments of quietude each day to sit in peace and silence, allowing your mind to settle and your thoughts to slowly fade away. Meditation is a practice of developing mindfulness and awareness, allowing you to watch your thoughts and feelings without judgement. By incorporating meditation into your daily routine, you can build greater resilience to stress and worry, allowing you to approach sexual situations with a sense of clarity and presence.

3. Mindfulness Techniques: Imagine tuning into your senses and fully immersing yourself in the present moment, enjoying the feelings and experiences as they unfold. Mindfulness methods involve paying attention to the here and now, without getting caught up in fears about the past or future. By adopting mindfulness during intimate meetings, you can improve your relationship with your partner and heighten your awareness of pleasurable sensations, leading to a greater sense of intimacy and happiness.

4. Progressive Muscle Calm: Picture yourself systematically tensing and relaxing each muscle group in your body, from your toes to your forehead, releasing stored stress and promoting

calm from head to toe. Progressive muscle relaxation is a method that involves alternating between tensing and relaxing different muscle groups, helping to ease physical tension and lower general stress levels. By practising progressive muscle relaxation regularly, you can train your body to recognize and release stress more effectively, allowing you to approach sexual situations with a greater sense of ease and comfort.

5. Visualization and Imagery: Imagine forming mental images of peaceful and calm settings, such as a relaxing beach or a lush forest, allowing yourself to engage in the sights, sounds, and feelings of these imagined landscapes. Visualisation and imaging methods involve conjuring up vivid mental pictures that evoke feelings of relaxing and calmness. By picturing yourself in peaceful settings, you can reduce stress and anxiety, allowing you to approach sexual situations with a greater sense of ease and confidence.

6. Guided Relaxation Scripts: Envision listening to a guided relaxation recording or following along with a written script that leads you through a number of relaxation routines, including deep breathing, progressive muscle relaxation, and

visualisation. Guided relaxation scripts provide organised direction for achieving a state of deep relaxation, helping you release tension and quiet the mind. By following along with a guided relaxation session, you can experience deep relaxation and stress relief, setting the stage for more enjoyable and fulfilling sexual encounters.

7. Journaling and Reflection: Picture yourself sitting down with a notebook and pen, allowing your thoughts and emotions to flow easily onto the page as you explore your feelings and experiences related to sexuality and intimacy. Journaling and reflection provide a chance for self-exploration and introspection, allowing you to identify and process underlying stresses and anxieties. By expressing your thoughts and feelings through writing, you can gain insight and perspective, lowering the mental burden of stress and anxiety and making space for greater intimacy and connection with your partner.

8. Social Support and Communication: Imagine calling out to trusted friends, family members, or a therapist to share your concerns and experiences related to rapid ejaculation and sexual performance anxiety. Social support and open conversation can be invaluable tools for dealing with stress and anxiety, giving validation,

empathy, and practical advice. By confiding in others and finding support, you can alleviate feelings of isolation and shame, creating a sense of connection and understanding that promotes mental well-being and resilience.

9. Self-Care Practices: Envision engaging in activities that feed and refresh your mind, body, and spirit, such as taking slow walks in nature, indulging in soothing baths, or performing gentle yoga or tai chi. Self-care practices are important for promoting general well-being and resilience, helping you recharge and rejuvenate after times of stress and anxiety. By prioritising self-care and making time for activities that bring you joy and relaxation, you can build resilience to stress and anxiety, improving your ability to handle sexual experiences with confidence and ease.

10. Aromatherapy: Imagine filling your space with the soothing smells of lavender, chamomile, or ylang-ylang essential oils, allowing their calming aromas to envelop you in a feeling of quiet and peace. Aromatherapy includes using essential oils drawn from aromatic plants to promote relaxation and reduce stress and worry. By diffusing relaxing essential oils or adding them to a warm bath, you can create a serene

environment that fosters relaxation and enhances your general sense of well-being.

11. Progressive Relaxation Apps: Envision getting a relaxing app on your smartphone or computer that offers guided meditation, deep breathing exercises, or progressive muscle relaxation sessions, allowing you to access relaxation methods whenever and wherever you need them. Progressive relaxation apps provide easy access to relaxation tools that can help you handle stress and anxiety on the go. By adding these apps into your daily routine, you can build resilience to stress and improve your ability to stay calm and centred during intimate meetings.

12. Biofeedback Training: Picture yourself using biofeedback devices or apps that track bodily signs of stress, such as heart rate variability or skin conductance, giving real-time feedback on your body's stress reaction. Biofeedback training involves learning to notice and regulate your body's physiological reactions to stress through visual or audio cues. By learning biofeedback methods, you can develop greater awareness and control over your stress levels, allowing you to manage your body's response to stressors and promote relaxation during intimate times.

13. Sexual Education and Counseling: Imagine getting advice from a trained sexual health educator or counsellor who can provide knowledge, support, and guidance on managing premature ejaculation and sexual performance anxiety. Sexual education and therapy meetings can help you gain a better understanding of the factors leading to premature ejaculation and develop coping strategies for beating performance anxiety. By addressing underlying psychological and emotional factors, you can build confidence and self-assurance in your sexual skills, leading to more enjoyable and fulfilling sexual experiences.

14. Cognitive-Behavioral Therapy (CBT): Envision participation in cognitive-behavioural therapy meetings with a trained therapist who can help you spot and question negative thought patterns and beliefs related to sexual performance and intimacy. CBT is a therapy method that focuses on changing dysfunctional ideas and behaviours through cognitive restructuring and behavioural strategies. By learning to reframe negative ideas and adopt more adaptive coping techniques, you can reduce performance anxiety and build trust in your ability to handle premature ejaculation, leading to better sexual satisfaction and well-being.

15. Acupuncture: Imagine undergoing acupuncture treatments, where thin needles are inserted into specific spots on the body to promote relaxing and balance energy flow. Acupuncture is an old Chinese healing technique that has been used for ages to alleviate stress, anxiety, and different health conditions. By engaging specific acupuncture points related to ease and sexual health, you can experience a reduction in performance anxiety and an improvement in sexual function.

16. Herbal Remedies: Envision studying herbal treatments that have been long used to promote relaxing and support sexual health. Herbs such as ashwagandha, ginseng, and horny goat weed have been used in traditional medicine systems for their adaptogenic and sexual qualities. By adding herbal supplements or teas into your daily routine, you may experience changes in stress resistance, sexual energy, and general well-being.

17. Sex Therapy: Picture engaging in sex therapy meetings with a qualified therapist who specialises in handling sexual concerns and dysfunctions. Sex therapy offers a supportive and non-judgmental place for people and couples

to discuss their sexual experiences, desires, and challenges. Through personalised therapy, education, and exercises, sex therapists can help you develop methods for managing premature ejaculation, enhancing intimacy, and better communication with your partner.

18. Breathwork Techniques: Imagine practising specific breathwork methods, such as the 4-7-8 breathing technique or the ujjayi breath, to create a state of relaxing and calmness. Breathwork involves conscious control and management of the breath to affect bodily and psychological states. By adding breathwork techniques into your daily routine or during intimate moments, you can regulate your nervous system, reduce stress hormones, and promote a feeling of relaxation and presence.

19. Erotic Sensate Focus Exercises: Envision acting in sensate focus exercises with your partner, where you take turns exploring each other's bodies in a non-sexual and sensual way. Sensate focus is a method used in sex therapy to improve intimacy, pleasure, and conversation between partners. By focusing on sensory experiences without the pressure of performance or orgasm, you can strengthen your relationship

with your partner, reduce anxiety, and boost
sexual pleasure.

20. Holistic Wellness Practices: Picture following
holistic health practices that promote balance
and harmony in mind, body, and spirit. Practices
such as yoga, tai chi, mindfulness meditation,
and reiki can help you develop a sense of inner
peace, strength, and energy. By incorporating
holistic health practices into your lifestyle, you
can support your general well-being and build a
basis for fulfilling and satisfying sexual
experiences.

By studying these additional stress management
methods, you can expand your collection of tools
for overcoming premature ejaculation and
promoting relaxation during intimate encounters.
Whether you're considering acupuncture or
herbal treatments, getting advice from a sex
therapist, practising breathwork techniques, or
accepting holistic wellness practices, each
method offers unique benefits that can contribute
to your sexual health and well-being.

By adding these stress management methods
into your daily routine, you can create a
supportive environment for overcoming
premature ejaculation and fostering closeness

and connection with your partner. Whether you're engaging in deep breathing exercises, meditation practices, mindfulness techniques, or progressive muscle relaxation, each method offers unique benefits that can help you handle sexual experiences with confidence and ease.

Chapter Three:

Natural Remedies and Techniques to Combat Premature Ejaculation: Unlocking the Power of Nature and Mind

Imagine a world where the keys to beating premature ejaculation are found not in a drugstore, but in the embrace of nature and the depths of the human mind. In this trip towards sexual health, we explore a realm of natural remedies and methods that offer hope and strength to those wanting to reclaim control over their sexual experiences.

Herbal supplements beckon us with promises of old knowledge and potent healing qualities. From the adaptogenic ability of ashwagandha to the aphrodisiac allure of ginseng, these botanical treasures hold the potential to return balance and energy to our intimate meetings. Through a deeper knowledge of herbal remedies and their effectiveness, we reveal the gentle yet profound ways in which nature's wealth can support our journey towards sexual pleasure.

But nature's healing touch goes beyond the world of plants and herbs. It reaches into the very core of our being, asking us to discover the power of breath and mindfulness. Breathing exercises and mindfulness methods offer pathways to inner calm and presence, allowing us to manage the storms of performance anxiety with grace and resilience. As we learn to harness the rhythm of our breath and develop mindful awareness, we find greater freedom and faith in our ability to accept intimacy with openness and joy.

And let us not forget the oft-neglected muscles of the pelvic floor, where strength and control hold the keys to continued pleasure. Pelvic floor movements, widely known as Kegels, offer a pathway to greater control and power over ejaculation. Through targeted exercises and mindful practice, we can awaken dormant muscles and build a deeper link to our body's innate knowledge, paving the way for enhanced sexual performance and happiness.

1. Exploring Herbal Supplements:
Imagine diving into the rich tapestry of herbal medicines, where old knowledge meets modern science in a harmonious mix of tradition and innovation. Herbal supplements offer a complete approach to treating premature ejaculation, harnessing the therapeutic qualities of plants to return balance and vigour to the body. From

tribulus terrestris to maca root, these botanical marvels hold the promise of improved sexual performance and longevity, free from the side effects often associated with synthetic medicines. By accepting the healing power of nature, we open ourselves to a world of possibility, where the gentle touch of herbs can guide us towards greater intimacy and satisfaction.

2. Embracing Breath and Mindfulness:
Picture yourself in a moment of quiet thought, as you tune into the rhythm of your breath and the feelings of the present moment. Breathing exercises and mindfulness methods offer a gateway to inner peace and present, allowing us to overcome the limits of performance anxiety and self-doubt. Through practices such as diaphragmatic breathing, box breathing, and mindfulness meditation, we learn to develop a sense of calm and centeredness that affects every part of our being. By harnessing the power of breath and awareness, we reclaim our agency and liberty in the world of intimacy, creating stronger connections with ourselves and our partners.

3. Empowering the Pelvic Floor:
Envision getting into the untapped potential of
the pelvic floor—the often-overlooked muscles
that hold the key to sexual control and energy.
Pelvic floor movements, generally known as
Kegels, offer a pathway to greater strength,
endurance, and awareness in the bedroom. By
participating in focused exercises that strengthen
the pelvic floor muscles, we can improve our
ability to delay ejaculation and prolong pleasure
during sexual activity. Through constant practice
and mindful attention, we can open the full
potential of our pelvic floor, empowering
ourselves to accept intimacy with confidence and
energy.

Join us as we start on a trip of discovery and
transformation, led by the wisdom of nature and
the resilience of the human spirit. Together, let
us explore the boundless potential of natural
remedies and methods to fight premature
ejaculation, reclaiming our sexual vigour and
accepting a future filled with desire, pleasure,
and possibility.

1. Exploring Herbal Supplements and Their Efficacy:

Imagine walking into a lively garden of ancient remedies, where the knowledge of generations past intertwines with the wonders of modern science. Here, amidst the rich foliage of nature's wealth, lies a treasure trove of herbal supplements, each brimming with the promise of renewed energy and sexual power.

Herbal supplements offer a holistic approach to addressing premature ejaculation, drawing upon the natural healing qualities of plants to address the root reasons of sexual dysfunction. Take, for example, tribulus terrestris, a plant famous for its ability to boost testosterone levels and improve desire. This plant powerhouse works in harmony with the body's natural processes, gently pushing it towards a state of balance and vigour.

Similarly, maca root, a hearty tuber native to the Andes mountains, has long been admired for its aphrodisiac qualities and stamina-enhancing effects. Rich in nutrients and adaptogenic chemicals, maca root acts as a natural tonic for the body and mind, revitalising energy levels and returning vigour to sexual encounters.

Unlike synthetic medicines, which often come with a laundry list of side effects and possible risks, herbal vitamins offer a softer, more harmonious approach to sexual health. By embracing the healing power of nature, we can tap into a wealth of botanical wonders that feed the body, mind, and spirit, paving the way for greater closeness and satisfaction in our relationships.

So, as you start on your journey towards sexual health, consider discovering the rich mix of herbal treatments that nature has to offer. From tribulus terrestris to maca root and beyond, these botanical partners stand ready to support you on your quest for improved sexual performance and endurance. Embrace the healing power of nature, and open the door to a world of possibility, where closeness and satisfaction await around every corner.

Here are some examples of herbal products widely used to treat premature ejaculation, along with their stated efficacy:

1. Tribulus Terrestris:
This plant, also known as puncture vine, is widely used in traditional medicine systems for its aphrodisiac qualities and ability to improve

sexual function. Tribulus terrestris is believed to boost libido, increase testosterone levels, and improve erectile function, making it a popular choice for individuals looking to address premature ejaculation.

2. Maca Root:
Maca root, native to the Andes mountains of Peru, has gained fame as a natural remedy for sexual problems. It is rich in nutrients and adaptogenic substances that support hormonal balance, energy levels, and sexual health. Maca root is believed to boost libido, improve sexual stamina, and enhance general sexual performance, making it a valuable partner in the treatment of premature ejaculation.

3. Ashwagandha:
Ashwagandha, also known as Indian ginseng, is an adaptogenic herb widely used in Ayurvedic medicine for its energising and aphrodisiac qualities. It is known to decrease stress and anxiety, improve sexual function, and increase fertility. Ashwagandha has been studied for its possible benefits in treating premature ejaculation by promoting relaxation and lowering performance anxiety.

4. Ginkgo Biloba:
Ginkgo biloba extract is produced from the leaves
of the ginkgo tree and has been used in
traditional Chinese medicine for ages. It is known
for its vasodilatory benefits, which improve blood
flow to the genitals and enhance sexual function.
Ginkgo biloba is believed to boost arousal,
improve erectile function, and delay ejaculation,
making it a popular choice for individuals wanting
natural treatments for premature ejaculation.

5. Horny Goat Weed:
Horny goat weed, also known as Epimedium, is
an ornamental plant native to China and other
parts of Asia. It has a long history of use in
traditional Chinese medicine for its aphrodisiac
qualities and ability to improve sexual
performance. Horny goat weed is believed to
increase libido, improve erectile function, and
prolong sexual intercourse, making it a hopeful
choice for individuals dealing with premature
ejaculation.

6. Saffron:
Saffron, the dried stigma of the Crocus sativus
flower, is one of the world's most expensive
spices and has been used for ages for its
medicinal qualities. It is known for its
mood-enhancing and libido-boosting benefits, as

well as its ability to improve sexual function. Saffron has been studied for its possible benefits in treating premature ejaculation by reducing anxiety and improving sexual satisfaction.

7. Ginseng:
Ginseng, especially Korean red ginseng, is a popular herb known for its adaptogenic properties and possible benefits for sexual health. It is thought to boost libido, improve erectile function, and increase stamina. Ginseng has been studied for its effects on sexual performance and premature ejaculation, with some studies showing that it may help delay ejaculation and improve overall sexual happiness.

8. Saw Palmetto:
Saw palmetto is a palm plant native to North America, widely used for its possible benefits for prostate health and urinary function. It is also thought to have aphrodisiac qualities and may support sexual health in men. While research on saw palmetto especially for premature ejaculation is limited, some personal evidence suggests that it may help improve sexual function and delay ejaculation in some people.

9. Yohimbe:

Yohimbe is obtained from the wood of the yohimbe tree, native to Central and West Africa. It contains an active compound called yohimbine, which is thought to have stimulant and aphrodisiac benefits. Yohimbe has been used traditionally to improve sexual ability and treat erectile dysfunction. Some people may find that yohimbe helps delay ejaculation and improve overall sexual pleasure, although it can also cause side effects and should be used with care.

10. Black Seed (Nigella Sativa):

Black seed, also known as Nigella sativa or black cumin, is a plant native to Southwest Asia. It has been used for ages in traditional medicine for its possible health benefits, including its purported aphrodisiac qualities. While research directly on black seed for premature ejaculation is limited, some studies show that it may have good benefits on sexual function and libido in men.

11. Damiana:

Damiana is a shrub native to Central and South America, widely used as an aphrodisiac and medicine for sexual health. It is believed to have mood-enhancing and libido-boosting benefits, making it a popular choice for individuals seeking natural treatments for sexual dysfunction. Some people may find that damiana helps improve sexual performance and delay ejaculation, although more study is needed to confirm its effectiveness for this purpose.

12. Tongkat Ali (Eurycoma longifolia):

Tongkat Ali, also known as Longjack, is a flowering plant native to Southeast Asia. It has a long history of use in traditional medicine for its aphrodisiac qualities and possible benefits for sexual health. Tongkat Ali is thought to raise testosterone levels, improve libido, and improve sexual performance. Some people may find that Tongkat Ali helps delay ejaculation and improve total sexual satisfaction.

13. Muira Puama:

Muira Puama, also known as strength wood, is a Brazilian shrub widely used as an aphrodisiac and tonic for sexual health. It is thought to boost libido, improve erectile function, and increase sexual energy. Muira Puama may help individuals having premature ejaculation by improving sexual desire and stretching the length of intercourse.

14. Cnidium Monnieri:

Cnidium Monnieri is a flowering plant native to China and other parts of Asia, widely used in Chinese medicine for its aphrodisiac effects and possible benefits for sexual health. It is thought to increase blood flow to the genitals, improve erectile function, and boost sexual ability. Cnidium Monnieri may help individuals dealing with premature ejaculation by promoting relaxation and increasing sexual energy.

15. Shilajit:

Shilajit is a sticky resin-like substance found in the Himalayan mountains, widely used in Ayurvedic medicine for its refreshing and aphrodisiac qualities. It is rich in minerals, fulvic acid, and other bioactive substances that support general health and vigour. Shilajit is thought to boost libido, improve sexual function, and increase stamina. Some people may find that Shilajit helps delay ejaculation and improve total sexual happiness.

These herbal products offer natural alternatives to pharmaceutical treatments for premature ejaculation, and many people report positive results when using them as part of a complete approach to sexual health. However, it's important to speak with a healthcare worker before starting any new supplement routine, especially if you have underlying health problems or are taking medicine.

Additionally, individual responses to herbal supplements may vary, so it's important to watch your body's reaction and change dose as needed.

2. Breathing Exercises and Mindfulness Techniques

Imagine a tranquil scene: you, sitting in a quiet place, focusing solely on the rhythm of your breath and the feelings of the present moment. This simple act of tuning into your breath is the basis of breathing exercises and mindfulness techniques—a strong tool in combating premature ejaculation.

Breathing exercises, such as diaphragmatic breathing and box breathing, invite you to connect with your breath deliberately. By taking slow, deep breaths from the diaphragm, you signal to your body that it's time to rest. Box breathing, where you inhale, hold, release, and hold again in equal counts, further calms the mind and body, promoting a state of rest and focus.

Diaphragmatic breathing, also known as deep belly breathing or abdominal breathing, is a simple yet effective method for combating premature ejaculation by promoting relaxation and lowering worry. Here's how diaphragmatic breathing works in basic terms:

1. Find a Comfortable Position:
Sit or lie down in an easy position, with your back straight and your shoulders loose.

2. Place Your Hand on Your Belly:
Place one hand on your belly, just below your ribs. This will help you feel the movement of your diaphragm as you breathe.

3. Inhale Slowly Through Your Nose:
Take a slow, deep breath in through your nose. As you breathe, picture your belly growing like a balloon, pushing your hand outwards. Try to fill your lungs fully with air.

4. Exhale Slowly Through Your Mouth: Release the breath slowly and evenly through your mouth. As you exhale, feel your belly deflate, and picture all the tightness and stress leaving your body with each breath.

5. Repeat:
Continue this pattern of slow, deep breathing for several minutes, focused on the rise and fall of your belly with each breath. Try to keep your breaths smooth and even, without any breaks or jerky moves.

By practising diaphragmatic breathing regularly, especially during times of worry or anxiety, you can train your body to rest more easily and control your arousal levels. This can help you keep control during intimate times and delay ejaculation, leading to longer-lasting and more satisfying sexual experiences.

Box breathing is a simple yet powerful method that can help fight premature ejaculation by promoting calm and managing arousal levels during intimate times. Here's how the process of box breathing works in basic terms:

1. Inhale:
Begin by taking a slow, deep breath in through your nose. Imagine filling your lungs with air like you're inflating a bubble. As you inhale, count to yourself quietly, counting to four as you breathe in. Picture the air filling up your chest and belly, growing softly.

2. Hold:
Once you've gotten a full breath in, hold your
breath for a count of four seconds. During this
break, try to keep your body relaxed and your
mind focused. Imagine holding onto that breath
like you're holding onto a valuable gift.

3. Exhale:
After keeping your breath, slowly exhale through
your mouth for another count of four seconds.
Imagine releasing all the tightness and worry
from your body as you breathe out. Feel your
chest and belly shrink as you let go of the
breath.

4. Hold Again:
Once you've emptied your lungs, pause for
another count of four seconds before taking your
next breath. This brief pause helps your body to
reset and prepare for the next wave of breathing.

5. Repeat:
Continue this process of inhaling for four
seconds, holding for four seconds, releasing for
four seconds, and holding again for four seconds.
Picture the breath moving around a square
shape, hence the name "box breathing."

By practising box breathing regularly, especially during times of closeness, you can train your body to stay cool and relaxed, even when faced with arousal or performance anxiety. This can help you delay ejaculation and lengthen the duration of sexual action, leading to more satisfying and enjoyable experiences for both you and your partner.

Mindfulness meditation takes this practice a step further, pushing you to notice your thoughts and sensations without judgement. As you develop awareness of the present moment, you begin to untangle yourself from the web of worries and concerns that often follow sexual encounters. Instead of getting lost in thoughts of performance or fear of premature ejaculation, you learn to centre yourself in the here and now, finding peace and acceptance in the present moment.

Through constant practice of these methods, you can rewire your body's reaction to sexual stimuli. Rather than responding impulsively to arousal, you develop a sense of calm and centeredness that allows you to handle intimate times with confidence and ease. By harnessing the power of breath and awareness, you reclaim control over your sexual experience, creating stronger bonds with yourself and your partner.

Here are some additional examples of breathing routines and mindfulness methods that can be used to fight premature ejaculation:
1. Deep Belly Breathing:
- Sit or lie down in a comfy position.
- Place one hand on your belly and the other on your chest.
- Inhale deeply through your nose, causing your belly to rise as you fill your lungs with air.
- Exhale slowly through your mouth, feeling your belly gently fall as you release the breath.
- Repeat this process for several minutes, focusing on the feeling of your breath moving in and out of your body.

2. 4-7-8 Breathing Technique:
- Sit or lie down easily and close your eyes.
- Inhale fully through your nose for a count of four seconds.
- Hold your breath for a count of seven seconds.

- Exhale slowly and fully through your mouth for a count of eight seconds.
- Repeat this pattern several times, allowing yourself to relax with each breath.

3. Mindfulness Meditation:
- Find a quiet place where you won't be disturbed and sit easily.
- Close your eyes and bring your attention to the feeling of your breath as it enters and leaves your body.
- Notice any thoughts, feelings, or sensations that arise without judgement, simply watching them as they come and go.
- If your mind wanders, slowly guide your attention back to your breath.
- Practise awareness meditation for a few minutes each day, gradually increasing the length as you become more comfortable with the practice.

4. Body Scan Meditation:
- Lie down in a comfortable position and close your eyes.
- Starting at your feet, bring your awareness to each part of your body, one at a time.
- Notice any tightness or pain in each area and actively relax those muscles as you exhale.
- Continue moving up through your body, checking each part from your feet to the top of your head.
- By the end of the body scan, you should feel more relaxed and settled in the present moment.

5. Visualisation Techniques:
- Close your eyes and picture yourself in a calm and peaceful setting, such as a serene beach or a quiet forest.
- Engage all your senses in the vision, noticing the sights, sounds, smells, and feelings around you.
- As you immerse yourself in these mental images, allow yourself to let go of any worry or tension you may be hanging onto.
- Visualise yourself feeling confident, relaxed, and in control during private times, free from worries about rapid ejaculation.

6. Alternate Nostril Breathing (Nadi Shodhana):
- Sit easily with your back straight and close your eyes.
- Use your right hand to close your right nose and inhale deeply through your left nostril.
- At the peak of your intake, close your left nose with your ring finger and exhale slowly through your right nostril.
- Inhale through your right nose, then close it and breathe through your left nostril.
- Repeat this pattern for several rounds, focusing on the smooth flow of breath and keeping a calm and steady pace.

7. Square Breathing:
- Visualise a square in your mind, and breathe
for a count of four as you trace the first side of
the square.
- Hold your breath for a count of four as you
trace the second side.
- Exhale for a count of four as you trace the third
side.
- Hold your breath again for a count of four as
you finish the square.
- Repeat this pattern for several rounds, keeping
a steady pace and focusing on the uniformity of
the square.

8. Progressive Muscle Relaxation (PMR):
- Begin by tensing the muscles in your feet as
much as you can, then slowly relax them as you
breathe.
- Gradually work your way up through your body,
tensing and relaxing each muscle group in turn,
including your legs, thighs, belly, chest, arms,
shoulders, neck, and face. - As you release
tightness from each muscle group, allow yourself
to sink deeper into relaxation, feeling the stress
melt away with each breath.

9. Counting Breath Meditation:
- Sit or lie down easily and close your eyes.

- Inhale deeply through your nose and quietly count "one" as you do so.
- Exhale slowly through your mouth and count "two" as you do so.
- Continue this process, adding up with each inhale and exhale, until you hit a count of ten.
- Start over at one and repeat the cycle for several rounds, focusing your attention on the flow of your breath and the act of counting.

10. Visualisation of Breath as Energy:
- Close your eyes and picture each breath as a flow of energy filling your body.
- Visualise this energy flowing throughout your body with each inhale, filling you with vigour and power.
- As you exhale, picture releasing any tension, worry, or negative feelings, letting them dissipate into the surrounding area.
- Continue this thought, feeling more relaxed and energised with each breath.

These examples show the variety of breathing exercises and mindfulness methods available to help people combat premature ejaculation and improve their sexual experience. Experiment with different techniques to find what works best for you, and add them into your daily routine for greatest benefit.

Embracing breath and awareness is not just about handling premature ejaculation—it's about reclaiming your power and control in the world of intimacy. It's about respecting the present moment, letting go of expectations, and enjoying the beauty of connection without fear or doubt. So, take a deep breath, and start on a journey of self-discovery and closeness that overcomes the limits of performance anxiety and self-doubt.

3. Pelvic Floor Exercises (Kegels) for Better Control.

Imagine finding a secret treasure chest within your own body—the pelvic floor muscles, often ignored but holding immense power when it comes to sexual control and stamina. Pelvic floor movements, like Kegels, are the key to unlocking this treasure trove, giving a pathway to greater strength, endurance, and awareness in the bedroom.

Picture this: with each squeeze and release of your pelvic floor muscles, you're building a base of sexual control. Just as a strong core supports your body in physical activities, a strong pelvic floor supports your sexual skills, allowing you to last longer and enjoy more satisfying intimacy.

By participating in focused workouts that specifically improve these muscles, you're investing in your sexual well-being. It's like giving your body a secret weapon—a hidden talent that only you possess. With constant practice and mindful attention, you can tap into this potential and change your sexual experiences.

So, how do you do it? It's as simple as squeezing and lifting the muscles around your pelvic area, as if you're trying to stop yourself from peeing halfway. Hold for a few seconds, then release and rest. Repeat this exercise regularly, gradually raising the length and strength of your contractions.

With each repeat, you're building your pelvic floor muscles, improving your ability to control ejaculation, and prolonging pleasure during sexual activity. You're becoming the master of your own sexual fate, inspired to accept intimacy with confidence and vitality.

Now, let's break it down further:

1. Find Your Pelvic Floor Muscles:
Before you can improve them, you need to identify your pelvic floor muscles. Imagine you're trying to stop yourself from passing gas or peeing midway. The muscles you engage to do this are your pelvic floor muscles.

2. Practise the Squeeze-and-Lift:
Once you've found your pelvic floor muscles, try squeezing and lifting them. Hold the tightness for a few seconds, then release and breathe. Aim for 10-15 repeats, gradually raising the length and strength of each contraction as you become more skilled.

3. Incorporate Into Your Routine:
Make pelvic floor exercises a normal part of your schedule, just like brushing your teeth or going for a jog. You can do them quietly anytime, anywhere—while sitting at your desk, watching TV, or even lying in bed.

4. Stay Consistent:
Like any workout program, consistency is key. Aim to practise Kegels daily, gradually raising the

number of repetitions and stopping times as your muscles become stronger.
5. Track Your growth: Keep a journal or use a tracking app to measure your Kegel movements and growth over time. Note any improvements in your ability to control ejaculation, as well as any changes in sexual pleasure and success.

6. Combine with Other Techniques: While Kegel exercises are strong on their own, they can be even more effective when paired with other techniques for fighting premature ejaculation. Consider adding relaxation techniques, conversation strategies with your partner, and lifestyle changes into your routine for a complete approach to better sexual energy.

7. Seek Professional help if Needed: If you're suffering to see results or have worries about your sexual health, don't hesitate to seek help from a healthcare professional or a qualified sex therapist. They can provide specific advice, direction, and support suited to your individual wants and circumstances.

With each repeat, you're strengthening your pelvic floor muscles and improving your control over ejaculation. You're taking care of your sexual health and well-being, encouraged to enjoy longer-lasting and more satisfying intimacy with your partner.

Remember, mastering Kegel exercises takes time and dedication, but the benefits in terms of better sexual performance and happiness can be well worth the effort. By investing in your pelvic floor health and taking proactive steps to handle premature ejaculation, you're investing in your general well-being and quality of life. So, accept the trip, stay consistent, and enjoy the benefits of empowered sexual confidence and energy.

So, accept the power of your pelvic floor, and unlock your full sexual potential. With Kegels as your secret weapon, you're on your way to a lifetime of satisfying and pleasurable sexual adventures.

Chapter Four:

Practical Tips for Bedroom Success: Elevating Intimacy and Performance

Welcome to a chapter tailored to improve your bedroom adventures like never before. If you're on a quest for practical, effective strategies to boost closeness and improve performance between the sheets, you're in the right place.

In this thorough guide, we'll explore a range of simple yet powerful techniques meant to revolutionise your time in the bedroom. From encouraging open communication with your partner to learning the art of sensate focus exercises, we'll uncover the secrets to building stronger bonds and maximising pleasure.

But that's not all. We'll also dive into proven techniques for prolonged arousal without losing happiness. By adding these natural remedies into your routine, you'll unlock the potential for longer-lasting, more fulfilling romance.

So, whether you're looking to reignite the flames of passion or take your bedroom game to the next level, join us on this journey to discover the practical tips that will change your bedroom success. It's time to improve your intimate moments and enjoy a deeper, more satisfying relationship with your partner.

Practical Tips for Bedroom Success

1. Conversation with Your Partner: Open and honest conversation is key to building closeness and understanding in the bedroom. Talk to your partner about your concerns, desires, and tastes, and work together to find answers that work for both of you.

2. Sensate Focus Exercises: Engage in sensate focus exercises to improve arousal and pleasure during private times. Focus on discovering each other's bodies through touch, without the pressure of performance or pleasure. This can help improve intimacy and sexual pleasure while lowering worry about premature ejaculation.

3. Techniques for Prolonging Arousal Without Ejaculation: Experiment with different methods for prolonged arousal without ejaculating, such as the stop-start technique or the squeeze technique. These methods involve briefly stopping or lowering stimulation when you feel

close to ejaculation, allowing you to regain control and delay climax.

By adding these simple and natural home remedies into your routine, you can fight premature ejaculation and enjoy more satisfying and fulfilling experiences in the bedroom with your partner.

1. Communication with Your Partner: The Foundation of Intimacy

Imagine your partnership as a garden. Just as a garden needs care, attention, and food to thrive, so does your link with your partner. And at the heart of this healthy relationship garden lies conversation – the soil from which intimacy and understanding bloom.

But what does conversation in the bedroom look like? It's more than just words; it's a dance of sensitivity, trust, and mutual respect. It's about expressing your wants and fears, listening to your partner's needs, and finding shared ground where both of you feel heard and respected.

So, how do you nurture this information garden? Start by making a safe place where honesty and openness can thrive. Share your thoughts, feelings, and dreams with your partner, knowing that they will be met with love and understanding.

But conversation isn't just about talking; it's also about listening – truly listening – to your partner's words, body language, and feelings. Pay attention to their cues, and show care and understanding in your answers.

And remember, conversation is a two-way street. Be receptive to feedback from your partner, and be ready to make adjustments to meet their wants and wishes. By supporting open and honest conversation in the bedroom, you lay the groundwork for deeper closeness, greater connection, and ultimately, more satisfying experiences together.

Imagine you and your partner as travellers, starting on a trip through the vast world of communication. Each talk is like a new path to find, filled with twists, turns, and secret treasures waiting to be unearthed.

As you explore this world together, remember to approach each exchange with curiosity and compassion. Be ready to explore new paths and

views, and accept the beauty of openness as you share your deepest thoughts and wishes.
But communication isn't just about giving; it's also about knowing. Take the time to truly listen to your partner, tuning in not only to their words but also to the feelings and goals behind them. Empathise with their experiences and validate their feelings, providing a safe place for them to express themselves openly and honestly.

And don't forget to enjoy the small wins along the way. Every moment of connection, every shared laugh, and every meaningful talk is a testament to the strength of your bond and the power of communication in your relationship.

So, as you continue your trip through the landscape of communication, remember to enjoy each step forward, knowing that with every word shared, you're building a stronger, more personal relationship with your partner.

Harnessing the Power of Communication to Combat Premature Ejaculation

Imagine the bedroom as a refuge where words flow like a gentle stream, creating a tapestry of closeness and understanding. In this sacred place, communication becomes a powerful tool in the fight against premature ejaculation, changing the way we feel pleasure and connection with our partners.

But how does conversation serve as a natural cure for premature ejaculation?
Let's dive into the details:

1. Setting the Stage: Before the curtains rise on the bedroom show, discussion lays the groundwork for success. By freely sharing your concerns and wishes with your partner, you create a supportive atmosphere where both of you feel empowered to address issues like premature ejaculation without judgement or shame.

2. Building Confidence: Just as a helpful crowd can embolden a performer on stage, open conversation in the bedroom can boost confidence and reduce performance nervousness. When you and your partner speak freely about your wants and expectations, you can approach intimacy with a sense of assurance, knowing that you're on the same page.

3. Exploring Solutions: Like master detectives solving a riddle, you and your partner can work together to explore possible solutions for

premature ejaculation. By brainstorming ideas, trying new techniques, and giving feedback to each other, you can discover what works best for both of you in overcoming this problem.

4. Sharing Duties: In the bedroom, conversation isn't just about talking – it's also about sharing duties. By involving your partner in the process of handling premature ejaculation, you spread the weight of the problem and improve your bond as a team. Together, you can handle the ups and downs of intimacy with honesty, understanding, and mutual support.

5. Celebrating Progress: Finally, conversation acts as a beacon of light, leading you through the darkness of premature ejaculation towards a better future. As you and your partner make steps in overcoming this challenge, enjoy your progress together. Acknowledge the small wins, show thanks for each other's efforts, and bask in the joy of shared closeness and connection.

6. Creating a Safe Space: Picture the bedroom as a refuge where weakness is welcomed and criticism is left at the door. Through open conversation, you and your partner create a safe place where you can share your fears, insecurities, and desires without fear of ridicule

or rejection. This safe haven allows you to dig deeper into the root causes of premature ejaculation and explore possible solutions together.

7. Experimenting with Techniques: Just as a scientist performs experiments to reveal new discoveries, you and your partner can try with different techniques to combat premature ejaculation. From trying new positions to adding mindfulness exercises into your lovemaking, conversation allows you to discuss what works and what doesn't, refining your approach until you find what brings you both the most pleasure and happiness.

8. Building Trust: Trust is the cornerstone of any good relationship, and conversation is the mortar that holds it all together. By freely discussing your experiences with premature ejaculation, you and your partner build trust and strengthen your relationship. This trust allows you to be open with each other, knowing that you will be met with understanding and support.

9. Strengthening Emotional Closeness: In the bedroom, emotional closeness is just as important as physical tenderness. Through conversation, you and your partner can improve

your emotional bond by sharing your inner thoughts, feelings, and wishes. This emotional link creates a strong base for intimacy and helps alleviate the pressure to perform, allowing you to rest and enjoy the moment without fear of judgement or judgement.

10. Cultivating Patience and Understanding: Like a plant that requires time and care to thrive, beating premature ejaculation requires patience and understanding. Through communication, you and your partner can develop these virtues as you manage the ups and downs of your sexual journey together. By being patient and understanding with each other, you create a helpful setting where growth and change can occur.

11. Encouraging Mutual Exploration: Think of the bedroom as a laboratory where you and your partner are free to explore and try without criticism. Through open conversation, you can support mutual discovery of each other's bodies and wants, finding new erogenous zones and methods that enhance pleasure and prolong arousal.

12. Setting Realistic Standards: Just as a navigator sets a path for a trip, conversation in the bedroom helps you to set realistic standards for your sexual experiences. By discussing what you both hope to achieve and recognizing that overcoming premature ejaculation is a process, not a quick fix, you can relieve pressure and create space for growth and improvement.

13. Addressing Emotional Causes: Premature ejaculation can often be linked to underlying emotional causes such as worry, anxiety, or past experiences. Through open dialogue, you and your partner can address these emotional triggers head-on, giving support and reassurance to each other as you manage the complexities of your sexual relationship.

14. Cultivating Erotic Imagination: The mind is a strong tool in the bedroom, capable of sparking passion and desire. Through conversation, you can develop your sexual imagination together, sharing dreams, desires, and role-playing situations that heighten arousal and lengthen pleasure.

15. Embracing Sexuality: Finally, conversation in the boudoir helps you to appreciate sexuality in all its forms. From speaking sweet nothings to

each other to engaging in sexual massage or tantric practices, you can strengthen your connection and closeness through the power of touch and conversation.

In essence, communication in the bedroom is not just about talking – it's about making a shared place where you and your partner can explore, experiment, and connect on a deeper level. By accepting open and honest communication, you can change your sexual experiences from mundane to magical, leaving behind the limitations of premature ejaculation and moving into a world of pleasure, passion, and deep intimacy.

2. Sensate Focus Exercises: Unlocking Intimacy and Pleasure

Imagine a dance of feelings, where touch becomes a language of its own, saying volumes of desire and connection. Sensate focus exercises ask you and your partner to start on a trip of exploration, using touch as a pathway to greater intimacy and pleasure. Let's dig into the details:

1. Setting the Scene:
Picture a dimly lit room decorated with soft candles and soothing music. This tranquil setting

produces the perfect mood for sensate focus exercises, allowing you and your partner to relax and connect on a deeper level.

2. Exploring Each Other's Bodies:
Begin by taking turns exploring each other's bodies with your hands, using gentle touches and strokes to awaken the senses. Focus on different areas of the body, from the nape of the neck to the soles of the feet, and pay attention to how your partner responds to each touch.

3. Heightening Sensations:
As you continue the exercise, try with different feelings to heighten arousal and pleasure. Try using feathers, silk scarves, or massage oils to add variety and energy to your touch. Encourage your partner to express their tastes and wants, creating a feedback loop of pleasure and exploration.

4. Removing the Pressure of Performance: One of the key benefits of sensate focus exercises is that they remove the pressure of performance and orgasm, allowing you to focus solely on the pleasure of the moment. By letting go of expectations and simply enjoying the feelings, you can reduce worry about premature

ejaculation and create a more relaxed and
fulfilling sexual experience.

5. Building Intimacy and Trust:
Sensate focus tasks promote a deeper sense of
intimacy and trust between you and your partner.
Through the shared experience of exploration
and discovery, you strengthen your emotional
link and develop your bond, paving the way for
more satisfying and fulfilling sexual encounters in
the future.

Sensate focus exercises offer a route to
heightened closeness, pleasure, and connection
in the bedroom. By embracing touch as a means
of communication, you and your partner can
overcome the limits of performance anxiety and
premature ejaculation, opening a world of
sensual joy and deep intimacy.

Sensate focus exercises serve as a natural
method to fight premature ejaculation by
treating both the physical and psychological parts
of the condition:

1. Reducing Performance Anxiety:
Sensate focus exercises create a relaxed
atmosphere where the focus is on discovery and
pleasure rather than performance or orgasm. By
removing the pressure to perform, people can

alleviate anxiety and stress associated with premature ejaculation, allowing them to enjoy sexual situations more fully.

2. Increasing Body Awareness:
Through sensate focus exercises, people become more sensitive to their own bodies and feelings, as well as those of their partners. This heightened awareness allows people to recognize the signs of approaching ejaculation and take steps to delay it, such as adjusting the pace or intensity of stimulation.

3. Enhancing Control:
Sensate focus exercises involve gradual development from non-genital to genital touch, allowing people to gradually build arousal and control over their sexual reactions. By practising mindful awareness and focusing on the present moment, people can learn to control their arousal levels and lengthen the time to ejaculation.

4. Improving Communication:
Engaging in sensate focus tasks requires open conversation between partners about wants, limits, and preferences. This conversation promotes trust, closeness, and understanding, providing a helpful atmosphere for addressing

problems related to premature ejaculation and working together to find answers.

5. Building Confidence:
As people become more comfortable with sensate focus exercises and find success in delaying ejaculation, their faith in their sexual skills grows. This improved confidence can have a good effect on general sexual functioning and happiness, reducing feelings of inadequacy or performance pressure.

6. Promoting Mindfulness:
Sensate focus activities urge people to be fully present in the moment, focusing their attention on the sensations of touch and pleasure. This mindfulness exercise helps people let go of distracting thoughts or fears about premature ejaculation, allowing them to experience sexual encounters with greater happiness and relaxation.

7. Strengthening Pelvic Floor Muscles: Sensate focus movements often involve gentle muscle twitches and relaxation methods, which can help strengthen the pelvic floor muscles over time. Stronger pelvic floor muscles are linked with better ejaculatory control, as they provide

support to the genitals and help manage the flow of semen during ejaculation.

8. Enhancing Emotional Connection: Engaging in sensate focus exercises promotes a stronger emotional connection between partners as they explore each other's bodies and share private moments of joy. This emotional link can help reduce stress and worry related to premature ejaculation, providing a helpful and understanding setting for both parties.

9. Developing Coping Strategies:
Through repeated practice of sensate focus routines, people can build coping techniques for controlling arousal and delaying ejaculation. These methods may include techniques such as stopping or changing stimulation patterns, using relaxation techniques, or focusing on pleasurable feelings in other parts of the body.

10. Long-Term Benefits:
Sensate focus workouts offer long-term benefits beyond just addressing premature ejaculation. They support intimacy, communication, and equal happiness in the relationship, leading to a healthier and more satisfying sexual connection overall. By incorporating these exercises into

their normal sexual practice, people can enjoy lasting gains in sexual function and pleasure.

11. Increasing Sexual Satisfaction:
Sensate focus exercises not only help in handling premature ejaculation but also contribute to total sexual pleasure. By focusing on the pleasure received from touch and discovery, people and their partners can experience heightened arousal and intimacy, leading to more satisfying sexual encounters.

12. Providing Non-Invasive Approach:
Unlike medications or invasive treatments, sensate focus movements offer a non-invasive and natural method to fighting premature ejaculation. This makes them approachable to individuals who prefer to avoid pharmaceutical interventions or medical procedures, offering a gentle and holistic option for better sexual function.

13. Customization for person Needs: Sensate focus exercises can be tailored to fit the unique needs and preferences of each person and their partner. Couples can try with different methods, levels of intimacy, and types of touch to find what works best for them, allowing for a

personalised approach to addressing premature ejaculation.

14. Encouraging Mutual Participation: Engaging in sensate focus activities requires active participation from both partners, promoting a sense of teamwork and mutual investment in sexual health and happiness. This shared experience improves the bond between partners and promotes a sense of teamwork in facing challenges related to premature ejaculation.

15. Empowering Self-Discovery:
Through sensate focus exercises, people have the opportunity to explore their own bodies and sexual reactions in a safe and helpful setting. This self-discovery can lead to greater self-awareness, confidence, and empowerment in one's sexuality, adding to general well-being and sexual fulfilment.

16. Enhancing Sensory Awareness:
Sensate focus exercises involve actively focusing on tactile feelings, which can heighten sensory awareness and sensitivity to touch. By giving close attention to the details of physical feelings, people can become more sensitive to their body's reactions and learn to better control arousal

levels, eventually helping in managing premature ejaculation.

17. Improving Sexual Self-Efficacy: Engaging in sensate focus exercises can boost individuals' confidence in their ability to control premature ejaculation and improve their sexual performance. As they gain skill in delaying ejaculation and pleasing their partner, their sexual self-efficacy improves, leading to a more positive view on their sexual abilities and relationships.

18. Supporting Relationship Dynamics: Incorporating sensate focus techniques into the sexual routine can improve the dynamics of the relationship. The collaborative and intimate nature of these tasks creates a stronger connection between partners, promotes empathy and understanding, and reinforces the idea of working together to solve difficulties, including premature ejaculation.

19. Encouraging Playfulness and Creativity: Sensate focus exercises provide a chance for couples to explore and experiment with different forms of touch and closeness in a fun and creative way. This sense of exploration and novelty can reignite desire and energy in the

relationship, making sexual encounters more enjoyable and satisfying for both parties.

20. Fostering Lasting Changes:
By regularly performing sensate focus routines, people can develop skills and strategies that can lead to lasting changes in their sexual behaviour and functioning. These exercises support a mindful and thoughtful approach to sexuality, setting the groundwork for better and more satisfying sexual experiences in the long run.

Sensate focus routines offer a holistic approach to treating premature ejaculation by boosting relaxation, body awareness, conversation, and confidence in the bedroom. By incorporating these movements into their sexual practice, people can experience greater control over their ejaculation and enjoy more fulfilling and satisfying sexual experiences with their partners.

3. Techniques for Prolonging Arousal Without Ejaculation: Mastering the Art of Control

Imagine going on a trip of self-discovery, where you learn the secrets to prolonging pleasure and avoiding satisfaction. Techniques for prolonging excitement without ejaculation offer a route to learning the art of control in the bedroom. Let's dig into the details:

1. The Stop-Start Technique: Picture a symphony director gracefully guiding the flow of music, knowing exactly when to pause and when to continue. The stop-start method involves noting the signs of impending ejaculation and briefly stopping all sexual stimulation. By taking a short stop, you give yourself time to cool down and regain control over your arousal levels before continuing.

2. The Squeeze Technique: Envision squeezing the brakes on a fast train, slowing down the motion just enough to stay on track. The squeeze method requires gently applying pressure to the base of the penis, just below the head, when you feel close to climax. This action briefly reduces blood flow to the penis, helping to delay ejaculation without fully stopping the sexual activity.

3. Mindful Awareness: Imagine being fully present in the moment, attuned to every feeling and detail of pleasure. Mindful awareness is a key component of learning methods for increasing arousal. By staying aware of your body's responses and arousal levels, you can preemptively engage before hitting the point of

no return, allowing you to extend the length of sexual activity without ejaculating prematurely.

4. Communication with Your Partner: Picture a dance between two partners, moving in perfect rhythm as they express their wants and limits. Effective communication with your partner is important when learning methods for prolonging arousal. Let them know when you need to pause or change the level of stimulation, and encourage them to provide feedback and support throughout the process.

5. Practice and Patience: Envision a sculptor shaping a beauty from a block of marble, carefully chiselling away until the perfect form emerges. Mastering methods for prolonged arousal takes practice and patience. Be ready to try with different methods and approaches, and don't be discouraged by failures along the way. With dedication and determination, you can gradually increase your stamina and control in the bedroom, leading to more enjoyable and fulfilling sexual experiences for both you and your partner.

6. Visualisation Techniques: Imagine controlling the power of your mind to control your body's response to arousal. Visualisation methods

involve mentally picturing calming scenes or diverting your focus away from sexual excitement when you feel yourself near ejaculation. By directing your thoughts towards relaxing images or engaging in mental distractions, you can successfully prolong arousal without ejaculating prematurely.

7. Edging: Picture walking along the edge of a cliff, teetering on the brink of climax but holding back just in time. Edging includes intentionally bringing yourself to the brink of orgasm multiple times during sexual action, then backing off before reaching the point of ejaculation. This method allows you to gradually build tolerance to high levels of arousal, extending the length of sexual encounters while keeping control over ejaculation.

8. Breathing Techniques: Envision the regular rise and fall of your chest as you breathe deeply and slowly, relaxing your body and mind. Breathing methods play a crucial role in controlling arousal and slowing ejaculation. By practising deep, diaphragmatic breathing during sexual activity, you can promote calm, reduce stress, and manage your heart rate, helping you

keep control over your arousal levels and avoid premature ejaculation.

9. Sensory Distraction: Imagine adding sensory distractions into your sexual experience, such as listening to music, focusing on tactile feelings, or incorporating different textures and temperatures into your surroundings. Sensory distractions can help shift your attention away from sexual excitement when you feel yourself getting too close to ejaculation, giving you the opportunity to prolong arousal and delay climax.

10. Positive Reinforcement: Picture praising your progress and wins along the way, acknowledging each small victory as you work towards overcoming premature ejaculation. Positive reinforcement involves noticing and rewarding yourself for successfully applying techniques for prolonging arousal without ejaculation. Whether it's a word of support from your partner, a pat on the back from yourself, or a small treat to celebrate your efforts, positive feedback can help reinforce your commitment to mastering control in the bedroom.

11. Pelvic Floor Exercises (Kegels): Visualise working the muscles of your pelvic floor, strengthening them like a fighter ready for

battle. Pelvic floor movements, also known as Kegels, involve tightening and calming the muscles that control urination and ejaculation. By performing Kegel movements regularly, you can improve your ability to control ejaculation and prolong arousal during sexual activity. Start by recognizing the muscles of your pelvic floor, then contract and hold them for a few seconds before relaxing. Gradually increase the length and volume of your contractions as you build strength and control over time.

12. Progressive Relaxation: Imagine stress melting away from your body like snow under the warmth of the sun. Progressive relaxation methods involve systematically tensing and then releasing different muscle groups in your body, promoting general relaxation and reducing stress that may contribute to premature ejaculation. By adding gradual relaxation into your pre-sexual practice, you can create a state of calm and readiness that improves your ability to prolong arousal and delay ejaculation.

13. Delay Sprays or Creams: Picture applying a thin layer of cream or spray to your penis, creating a brief barrier that lowers sensitivity and slows ejaculation. Delay sprays or creams contain chemicals like lidocaine or benzocaine,

which numb the nerve ends in the penis and lengthen the time it takes to reach climax. By using these items as recommended, you can successfully delay ejaculation and extend the length of sexual activity, providing greater happiness for you and your partner.

14. Anaesthetic Condoms: Envision slipping on a condom that not only offers security but also prolongs joy. Anaesthetic condoms are coated with a mild numbing drug, such as benzocaine, which lowers sensitivity and slows ejaculation. By using anaesthetic condoms during sexual activity, you can prolong arousal and extend the length of intercourse without losing feeling or pleasure.

15. Sexual Positions: Picture trying different sexual positions that allow for greater control and energy in the bedroom. Certain sexual positions, such as those that involve less entry depth or allow for slower, more controlled movements, can help delay ejaculation and lengthen sexual activity. Experiment with various positions to find what works best for you and your partner, and don't be afraid to get artistic and adventurous in your discovery.

16. Distraction Techniques: Imagine redirecting your attention away from sexual feelings when

you feel yourself nearing ejaculation, successfully delaying climax. Distraction methods involve mentally moving your attention to non-sexual thoughts or actions during intimate times. This could include counting backwards from a high number, repeating a song in your head, or visualising a calming scene. By engaging in distraction methods, you can briefly suppress arousal and lengthen the period of sexual activity without ejaculating prematurely.

17. Sexual dreams: Envision exploring romantic dreams or scenes in your mind during sexual activity, increasing arousal while simultaneously delaying ejaculation. Sexual dreams can serve as a form of mental stimulation that improves arousal and prolongs sexual pleasure. By indulging in your dreams, you can keep a heightened state of arousal without reaching the point of climax too fast, allowing for longer-lasting and more satisfying sexual experiences.

18. Tantric Techniques: Picture adding tantric principles into your sexual practice, focusing on prolonging pleasure and achieving greater levels of closeness with your partner. Tantric methods stress awareness, breathwork, and energetic connection during sexual action, allowing for

heightened feelings and longer arousal. By
learning and performing tantric methods, you
can develop a more holistic approach to sexuality
that prioritises pleasure, connection, and life in
the bedroom.

19. Scheduled Masturbation: Imagine putting
aside specific time for masturbation, using it as a
chance to practise techniques for slowing
ejaculation and increasing sexual energy.
Scheduled masturbation involves actively
stimulating yourself to the point of arousal
without ejaculating, then stopping or lowering
stimulation before climax. By learning
self-control and arousal management during
single sexual activity, you can develop greater
control over your ejaculatory response and
improve your performance during partnered sex.

20. Sexual Mindfulness: Envision approaching
sexual action with a sense of mindfulness and
presence, fully immersing yourself in the feelings
and experiences of the moment. Sexual
mindfulness involves being fully aware of your
body, your partner, and the surroundings during
private moments, allowing for greater connection
and heightened joy. By developing sexual
awareness, you can reduce performance anxiety,

increase arousal control, and lengthen the period
of sexual activity without ejaculating soon.

Chapter Five:

Creating a Sustainable Plan

In the quest for beating premature ejaculation, starting on a sustainable journey is key to long-lasting success. It's not just about quick fixes or temporary solutions but rather about crafting a personalised plan that meets individual needs and promotes permanent change. By setting realistic goals and tracking progress along the way, individuals can stay inspired and focused on their trip towards better sexual performance. Moreover, incorporating long-term strategies guarantees that the progress made is kept over time, paving the way for a happy and satisfying sex life. So, let's dig into the art of making a sustainable plan to fight premature ejaculation, enabling individuals to take charge of their sexual health and unlock a world of pleasure and happiness.

In this journey towards overcoming premature ejaculation, it's important to understand that there's no one-size-fits-all answer. Each person is unique, with different wants, preferences, and difficulties. Therefore, creating a personalised method is paramount. By adapting strategies and techniques to fit specific situations, people can address root causes and find solutions that work best for them.

Setting realistic goals is another crucial aspect of making a sustainable plan. Instead of looking for instant transformation, it's important to break down the trip into manageable steps and celebrate progress along the way. By acknowledging successes, no matter how small, people can stay motivated and committed to their goals.

Moreover, tracking progress helps people to identify what's working well and where changes may be needed. Whether it's keeping a journal, using tracking apps, or getting feedback from a partner, monitoring success offers useful insights into the effectiveness of different strategies.

Lastly, incorporating long-term strategies guarantees that changes in sexual ability are kept over time. This involves not only implementing techniques to handle current concerns but also adopting healthy lifestyle habits and conversation practices that support ongoing sexual wellness.

By adopting a personalised, goal-oriented, and sustainable approach, individuals can beat premature ejaculation and develop a happy and enjoyable sex life that lasts a lifetime.

This trip toward overcoming premature ejaculation is not just about reaching a goal; it's about adopting a lifestyle that supports sexual health and fulfilment. By creating a sustainable plan, people can create lasting changes that positively impact their general well-being and relationships.

One important part of this journey is learning that growth may not always be linear. There may be setbacks and challenges along the way, but these moments provide important chances for learning and growth. By staying resilient and committed to the process, people can navigate through hurdles and continue going forward toward their goals.

Additionally, getting help and advice can be instrumental in keeping momentum and staying on track. Whether it's through therapy, support groups, or trusted healthcare workers, having a supportive network can provide motivation and useful insights throughout the trip.

Ultimately, building a sustainable plan to fight premature ejaculation is about allowing people to take control of their sexual health and well-being. By accepting personalised strategies, making realistic goals, tracking progress, and adding long-term solutions, individuals can start on a journey toward a more fulfilling and satisfying sex life, one step at a time.

1. Developing a Personalised Approach Based on Individual Needs.

When it comes to fighting premature ejaculation, there is no one-size-fits-all answer. Each individual's experience with premature ejaculation is unique, affected by various factors such as physical health, psychological well-being, relationship interactions, and lifestyle habits. Therefore, developing a personalised method tailored to individual needs is important for successfully addressing and managing premature ejaculation.

1. Assessment and Understanding: The first step in creating a personalised method is to measure and understand the underlying factors leading to premature ejaculation. This may involve reviewing physical health, such as finding any underlying medical problems or hormonal

imbalances. Additionally, knowing psychological factors such as worry, anxiety, and past experiences can provide useful insights into the root reasons of premature ejaculation.

2. Identifying Triggers and Patterns: Once the underlying factors are found, it's important to identify triggers and patterns unique to the person. This may involve keeping a log to track episodes of premature ejaculation, noting any common causes such as certain sexual positions, stresses, or relationship dynamics. By finding patterns, people can gain a better understanding of their unique obstacles and create targeted strategies to meet them.

3. Exploring Treatment choices: With a clear understanding of the underlying factors and triggers, people can explore various treatment choices geared to their unique needs. This may include lifestyle modifications, such as dietary changes, regular exercise, and stress management methods, which can have a significant effect on sexual health and function. Additionally, people may consider therapy or coaching to address psychological factors leading to premature ejaculation and learn coping techniques to handle stress and worry.

4. Implementing Behavioural Techniques: Behavioural techniques, such as the start-stop method, squeeze technique, and pelvic floor movements (Kegels), can be successful in improving ejaculatory control and prolonging sexual activity. These methods focus on improving awareness and control over the body's responses to sexual stimulation, allowing people to delay ejaculation and improve sexual satisfaction for both partners.

5. discussion and Partner Involvement: Finally, building a personalised method to fighting premature ejaculation involves open and honest discussion with sexual partners. Partners can play a supportive part in the process by providing understanding, motivation, and feedback. Collaboratively exploring and trying with different techniques and strategies can improve closeness and enhance the success of treatment efforts.

6. Holistic Approach: Taking a holistic approach includes considering all aspects of one's life that may lead to premature ejaculation. This includes physical health, mental well-being, emotional state, and living factors. By handling these areas thoroughly, people can create a more balanced and supportive setting for controlling premature ejaculation.

7. Individualised Strategies: No two people are alike, so it's crucial to develop strategies that are tailored to each person's unique wants and preferences. This may involve trying with different techniques, treatments, and lifestyle changes to find what works best for them. For example, while some people may benefit from relaxation methods like meditation or yoga, others may find success with specific workouts or dietary changes.

8. Trial and Error: Finding the most effective way to fight premature ejaculation often involves some trial and error. It's important for people to be patient and persistent as they study different strategies and methods. What works for one person may not work for another, so it's important to stay open-minded and adaptable throughout the process.

9. Regular Evaluation and Adjustment: As people improve on their journey to combat premature ejaculation, it's important to regularly assess their approach and make adjustments as needed. This may involve tracking progress, reassessing goals, and getting additional help or advice when appropriate. By staying proactive and invested in

the process, people can continue to refine their method and optimise their results over time.

10. Long-Term Maintenance: Finally, keeping growth and avoiding relapse takes ongoing effort and dedication. Individuals should continue to incorporate successful strategies and habits into their daily routine to sustain gains in ejaculatory control and sexual happiness. This may include keeping a healthy lifestyle, practising stress management methods, and nurturing good conversation and intimacy with sexual partners.

11. Integration of Support Systems: Incorporating support systems into the personalised method can provide additional tools and motivation along the way. This may involve getting advice from healthcare professionals, such as urologists, sex therapists, or psychologists, who specialise in sexual health and problems. Support groups or online communities can also offer a feeling of camaraderie and validation, allowing people to share experiences, insights, and tips with others facing similar difficulties.

12. Mind-Body Connection: Recognizing the connection of mind and body is important in building a holistic approach to fighting premature

ejaculation. Practices such as mindfulness meditation, relaxation methods, and body awareness exercises can help people develop a better understanding of their physical feelings and mental reactions during sexual activity. By fostering a more conscious and present awareness, people can gain greater control over their ejaculatory reflex and improve their overall sexual experience.

13. Exploration of sexuality: Embracing sexuality and pleasure beyond the goal of ejaculation can change the focus from performance to connection and closeness. Encouraging study of sensual touch, erogenous zones, and non-genital stimulation can expand the range of sexual experiences and ease pressure to achieve a specific result. By fostering a sense of curiosity and playfulness in the bedroom, people can create a more relaxed and enjoyable approach to sexual activity, lowering anxiety and performance-related stress.

14. Education and Empowerment: Educating oneself about the physiology of ejaculation, sexual response cycles, and common beliefs surrounding premature ejaculation can encourage people to take an active part in their sexual health. Understanding how factors such as

arousal levels, stimulation methods, and psychological state affect ejaculatory control can help decision-making and improve self-awareness during sexual experiences. By becoming informed champions for their own sexual well-being, people can navigate obstacles with confidence and assertiveness, seeking out resources and strategies that fit with their values and preferences.

15. Celebration of Progress: Celebrating milestones and successes along the road to beating premature ejaculation can provide motivation and support to continue forward. Whether it's noting changes in ejaculatory control, greater closeness with a partner, or personal growth in self-awareness and confidence, admitting progress promotes a sense of success and supports positive habits. By taking time to honour and enjoy wins, individuals can develop grit and perseverance in their efforts to achieve their sexual health goals.

By creating a personalised method based on individual needs, people can successfully handle and control premature ejaculation, eventually improving their overall sexual health and well-being. With patience, determination, and a desire to explore and adapt, people can achieve lasting success in their efforts to fight premature ejaculation and improve their sexual pleasure.

2. Setting Realistic Goals and Tracking Progress.

Setting realistic goals and tracking progress are important components of any trip towards overcoming premature ejaculation. By setting clear objectives and monitoring one's progress, individuals can maintain focus, stay inspired, and make informed adjustments to their approach as required. Here's a better look at how setting goals and tracking progress can ease the process:

1. Define Clear Objectives: Begin by defining specific, realistic goals linked to controlling premature ejaculation. These goals should be achievable, measurable, and important to the individual's wants and circumstances. For example, a goal might be to increase the length of sexual action without ejaculating prematurely by a certain percentage within a defined timeframe.

2. Break Down Goals Into Smaller Steps: Break down large goals into smaller, more doable steps or milestones. This allows for incremental

progress and stops people from feeling overwhelmed or disheartened by the magnitude of the final goal. Each step should be doable within an acceptable time frame and add to the general goal of handling premature ejaculation.

3. Establish a schedule: Set a schedule for achieving each step or milestone, taking into account factors such as personal tastes, lifestyle responsibilities, and the seriousness of premature ejaculation. While some people may improve quickly, others may require more time and patience. It's important to be flexible and change timelines as needed to suit individual wants and circumstances.

4. Identify Monitoring Tools: Determine how success will be tracked and watched over time. This may involve keeping a log or diary to record sexual experiences, including factors such as length of intercourse, perceived levels of arousal, and any methods or strategies applied to control premature ejaculation. Alternatively, people may use specific apps or online platforms created for tracking sexual health and performance.

5. Regularly Assess Progress: Regularly assess progress towards set goals, using the identified tracking tools to track changes and trends over

time. This allows people to spot patterns, notice areas of improvement, and pinpoint any challenges or setbacks that may arise along the way. By staying involved and proactive in monitoring progress, people can keep momentum and stay focused on their goals.

6. Celebrate Achievements: Celebrate achievements and goals made along the journey to managing premature ejaculation. Acknowledge progress, no matter how small, and enjoy wins as proof of personal growth and Improvement. This positive feedback can boost drive, confidence, and resilience, inspiring individuals to continue their efforts and beat any hurdles met along the way.

7. Adjust Goals and Strategies as Needed: Be willing to change goals and tactics based on ongoing feedback and review of progress. If certain methods or approaches are not yielding the desired results, explore alternative options and change the plan accordingly. Flexibility and willingness to experiment are key to finding what works best for each individual's unique situations and tastes.

8. Seek Professional Guidance: In cases where managing premature ejaculation proves difficult, getting professional guidance can provide useful

support and knowledge. Consulting with a healthcare provider, such as a urologist, sex therapist, or psychologist, can offer specific suggestions, diagnostic tests, and evidence-based treatments geared to individual needs. These professionals can provide insights into underlying factors leading to premature ejaculation, give advice on effective treatment choices, and support people in developing complete strategies for long-term success.

9. Utilise Technology: Take advantage of technological developments to help in goal setting and progress tracking. Mobile apps, wearable devices, and online platforms created for sexual health and fitness can provide engaging tools, educational resources, and personalised feedback to support people in managing premature ejaculation. These digital solutions offer convenience, accessibility, and anonymity, allowing people to receive help and resources from the comfort of their own home.

10. Engage in Peer Support: Participate in peer support groups or online communities focused on sexual health and rapid ejaculation. Connecting with others who share similar experiences can provide support, motivation, and useful tips for handling premature ejaculation. Peer support

offers a sense of unity and understanding, reducing feelings of isolation and shame while creating a helpful environment for learning, growth, and mutual strength.

11. Practice Self-Compassion: Cultivate self-compassion and kindness towards oneself throughout the process of controlling premature ejaculation. Recognize that setbacks and difficulties are a normal part of the process and treat oneself with kindness, understanding, and acceptance. Practice self-care activities that encourage relaxation, stress reduction, and mental well-being, such as mindfulness meditation, physical exercise, and artistic expression. By nurturing oneself with kindness and self-care, people can build grit, confidence, and inner strength to manage the ups and downs of overcoming premature ejaculation.

12. Celebrate Progress, Not Perfection: Shift the focus from reaching perfection to honouring progress and growth along the way. Recognize that managing premature ejaculation is a journey, not a goal, and welcome each step forward as a testament to personal grit and drive. Embrace the lessons learned from both wins and failures, and use them as chances for reflection, learning, and growth. By choosing an

attitude of progress over perfection, individuals can develop resilience, optimism, and a sense of empowerment in their efforts to handle premature ejaculation and improve their overall sexual well-being.

13. Explore Alternative treatments: Consider exploring alternative treatments and holistic techniques that may support standard methods for handling premature ejaculation. Practices such as acupuncture, herbal medicine, aromatherapy, and yoga have been used for ages to support general health and well-being, including sexual health. While study on the usefulness of these therapies especially for premature ejaculation may be limited, some people find relief and benefit from incorporating these practices into their holistic health routine.

14. Maintain Overall Health and Wellness: Prioritise overall health and wellness as essential components of handling rapid ejaculation. Adopting a healthy lifestyle that includes regular physical exercise, good diet, adequate sleep, and stress management can contribute to better sexual function and energy. Addressing underlying health problems, such as obesity, diabetes, and hypertension, can also help ease factors leading to premature ejaculation. By

taking a holistic approach to health and wellness, people can optimise their general well-being and enhance their sexual success and happiness.

15. Educate Yourself: Educate yourself about rapid ejaculation, its causes, signs, and treatment choices. Knowledge empowers people to make informed choices about their sexual health and seek suitable help and tools. Stay updated on study results, evidence-based treatments, and new therapies for controlling premature ejaculation. Engage in ongoing learning and conversation with healthcare providers, trusted sources, and respected groups specialising in sexual health and wellness. By becoming educated advocates for their own sexual health, people can play an active part in managing premature ejaculation and achieving optimal sexual satisfaction and well-being.

16. Address Relationship Dynamics: Consider the role of relationship dynamics in controlling premature ejaculation. Open and honest conversation with partners about sexual wants, desires, and worries can promote understanding, trust, and closeness. Explore ways to improve mental connection, closeness, and shared pleasure within the relationship. Address any underlying relationship problems or conflicts that

may add to stress, anxiety, or performance pressure. By nurturing healthy and helpful relationships, people can create a conducive environment for controlling premature ejaculation and creating satisfying sexual experiences for both partners.

17. Stay Positive and Persistent: Maintain a positive attitude and continue in your efforts to handle premature ejaculation. Understand that success may take time, and setbacks are a natural part of the process. Stay committed to your goals, and believe in your ability to beat obstacles and achieve success. Draw inspiration from your successes, no matter how small, and use them as fuel to continue going forward. With drive, resilience, and a positive mindset, you can successfully handle premature ejaculation and enjoy fulfilling and satisfying sexual experiences.

By setting realistic goals, breaking them down into doable steps, establishing a schedule, watching progress, praising successes, and changing strategies as needed, individuals can effectively track their journey towards controlling premature ejaculation. This organised method promotes responsibility, motivation, and confidence, eventually leading to greater success in beating premature ejaculation and improving overall sexual pleasure and well-being.

3. Incorporating Long-term Strategies for Maintaining Improved Performance.

Incorporating long-term strategies for keeping better performance involves making sustainable lifestyle changes, developing healthy habits, and nurturing ongoing self-care practices to support sexual health and well-being. These strategies aim to not only address the immediate concerns related to premature ejaculation but also promote long-lasting changes in sexual function and happiness. Here are some key methods to consider:

1. Consistent Practice: Consistency is important when adopting methods to combat premature ejaculation. Whether it's learning relaxation techniques, engaging in pelvic floor exercises, or studying sensate focus exercises, commit to adding these practices into your daily routine. Consistent practice helps you to reinforce good habits, build resilience, and eventually improve your sexual ability over time.

2. Holistic Wellness: Take a holistic approach to wellness by tackling all parts of your health,

including physical, mental, social, and relational factors. Maintain a healthy lifestyle that values regular exercise, nutritious food, adequate sleep, and stress management methods. Attend to your general well-being to support optimal sexual health and success in the long run.

3. Mindful Sexual Practices: Cultivate awareness and presence during sexual meetings to improve pleasure, intimacy, and control. Practice mindfulness methods, such as deep breathing, body scanning, and sensory awareness, to stay present and linked with your partner during private times. By focusing on the feelings and experiences in the present moment, you can reduce performance anxiety, prolong arousal, and improve total sexual happiness.

4. Open Communication: Foster open and honest conversation with your partner about sexual wants, tastes, and concerns. Create a safe and loving place for talking closeness and handling any challenges related to premature ejaculation. Collaborate with your partner to discover new techniques, try with different strategies, and find answers that work best for both of you. Effective conversation improves emotional connection, builds trust, and enhances sexual pleasure in the long run.

5. Regular Check-ins: Schedule regular check-ins with yourself and your partner to assess success, find areas for change, and adjust your method as needed. Reflect on your experiences, wins, and challenges in handling premature ejaculation, and brainstorm new strategies or changes to your current routine. Regular check-ins help you stay responsible, track your progress, and keep momentum towards your long-term goals.

6. Continued Education: Stay Informed about improvements in sexual health studies, treatment choices, and tools for handling premature ejaculation. Seek out reliable sources of information, attend classes or seminars, and stay involved in ongoing learning opportunities related to sexual health. By staying educated and informed, you can make informed choices, fight for your sexual health needs, and receive the support and resources necessary for keeping improved sexual performance in the long run.

7. Explore Pleasurable Techniques: Continuously explore and try with different sexual techniques and positions that can help delay ejaculation and improve pleasure for both partners. Encourage open conversation with your partner to identify

what feels most enjoyable and beneficial to continuing sexual activity.

8. Practise Sensory Awareness: Develop heightened sensory awareness during sexual situations by tuning into the feelings and feedback from your body. Pay attention to subtle cues of arousal and approaching climax, allowing you to change stimulation and pacing properly to lengthen the experience.

9. Strengthen Emotional relationship: Prioritise emotional intimacy and relationship with your mate outside of the bedroom. Engage in activities that promote emotional bonding, such as shared hobbies, important talks, and expressions of love. A strong emotional link can build a supportive base for addressing sexual challenges and keeping overall relationship happiness.

10. Seek Professional Support: Consider getting advice from a trained healthcare professional or sex therapist who specialises in sexual health and intimacy problems. A trained professional can provide personalised assessment, advice, and treatment choices geared to your unique wants and situations. Therapy sessions can offer useful insights, tactics, and support for managing

premature ejaculation and improving sexual happiness in the long run.

11. Manage Performance Pressure: Challenge false standards and social demands linked to sexual performance. Focus on enjoying the trip of sexual discovery and intimacy with your partner, rather than fixating on achieving specific performance goals. Cultivate an attitude of acceptance, self-compassion, and sexual self-confidence, realising that sexual experiences are dynamic and can vary from one meeting to another.

12. Practice Self-Care: Prioritise self-care techniques that encourage relaxation, stress relief, and general well-being. Engage in activities that help you relax and recover, such as mindfulness meditation, yoga, or spending time in nature. Managing stress and prioritising self-care can help ease performance anxiety and add to a more enjoyable and fulfilling sexual experience.

13. enjoy Progress: Acknowledge and enjoy the progress you make in handling premature ejaculation and improving sexual performance. Celebrate accomplishments, no matter how small, and praise your efforts and successes

along the way. Positive reinforcement can boost motivation, confidence, and resilience in overcoming obstacles and keeping long-term gains in sexual performance and happiness.

14. Healthy Sleep Habits: Prioritise excellent sleep as part of your general health routine. Aim for regular sleep schedules, build a relaxing bedtime routine, and ensure your sleep surroundings are suitable for restorative rest. Quality sleep supports hormonal balance, mood control, and general well-being, which can positively affect sexual function and performance.

15. Limit Alcohol and Substance Use: Moderation in alcohol consumption and avoidance of recreational drugs can help mitigate factors that contribute to premature ejaculation, such as altered reasoning, decreased libido control, and reduced sexual response. Opt for healthier options and be aware of how drugs affect your sexual experiences and function.

16. Maintain Sexual Variety: Embrace diversity and surprise in your sexual experiences to keep things fresh and exciting. Explore different places, scenes, and activities that appeal to you and your partner's interests and fantasies.

Variety can help avoid boredom, reduce performance pressure, and improve total sexual pleasure and closeness.

17. Regular Physical Examinations: Schedule regular check-ups with your healthcare provider to watch your general health and address any underlying medical conditions that may impact sexual function. Discuss any worries or symptoms linked to premature ejaculation openly with your doctor to discuss possible causes and treatment choices.

18. Practice Patience and Persistence: Recognize that controlling premature ejaculation is a journey that may take time, patience, and consistent effort. Be patient with yourself and your partner as you handle challenges and setbacks along the way. Stay committed to your goals, persevere through hurdles, and keep a positive attitude towards your progress and growth.

19. Embrace Sexual Education: Educate yourself and your partner about sexual health, anatomy, and joy to improve your understanding and respect of each other's bodies and wants. Learn about sexual techniques, communication skills, and intimacy-building methods that can improve

your sexual experiences and foster mutual satisfaction.

20. Cultivate Gratitude and Connection: Cultivate gratitude for the gift of closeness and connection with your partner. Express respect for each other's presence, efforts, and gifts to your relationship and sexual experiences. Cultivating gratitude and connection strengthens emotional bonds, creates resilience, and increases the quality of your sexual exchanges and overall relationship happiness.

By incorporating these long-term strategies into your lifestyle and relationship dynamics, you can successfully control premature ejaculation and enjoy sustained changes in sexual function, happiness, and general well-being over time. Remember that consistency, mindfulness, conversation, and ongoing self-care are important components of keeping long-lasting changes in sexual function and intimacy.

Conclusion:

In conclusion, "Premature No More: Simple and Natural Home Remedies to Combat Premature Ejaculation for Improved Performance" offers a complete approach to handling premature ejaculation and improving sexual performance through simple and natural methods. Throughout this guide, we've covered a variety of strategies and techniques aimed at empowering men to take control of their sexual health and happiness.

From understanding the causes and effects of premature ejaculation to making lifestyle changes, adding herbal supplements, and practising awareness and communication skills, each part of our discussion has added to a complete approach to controlling premature ejaculation.

Key points and tactics covered include:

1. Understanding Premature Ejaculation:
We dug into the meaning, common causes, and effects of premature ejaculation, dispelling myths and misconceptions along the way. By getting a greater knowledge of this situation, people can better navigate its challenges and seek appropriate solutions.

2. Natural Remedies and Techniques:
We studied a range of natural treatments and techniques, including dietary changes, exercise and physical activity, stress management, herbal supplements, sensory focus exercises, and methods for prolonging arousal without ejaculation. These methods offer accessible and sustainable alternatives to pharmaceutical treatments, supporting general health and well-being.

3. Practical Tips for Bedroom Success:
We stressed the importance of conversation with partners, sensate focus exercises, and techniques for prolonged arousal as practical strategies for improving closeness and pleasure in the bedroom. By fostering open conversation and enjoying pleasurable experiences together, couples can improve their connection and happiness.

4. Creating a Sustainable Plan:
We emphasised the importance of creating a personalised approach based on individual needs, setting reasonable goals, tracking progress, and incorporating long-term strategies for keeping better performance. By adopting a sustainable plan tailored to their unique situations, people

can achieve lasting results and enjoy fulfilling
sexual experiences.

"Premature No More" serves as a complete
resource for men wanting easy and natural
solutions to fight premature ejaculation and
improve their sexual performance. By following
the strategies and techniques described in this
guide, individuals can reclaim control over their
sexual health, foster greater intimacy with their
partners, and enjoy a more satisfying and
fulfilling sex life.

As you start on this road towards better
performance and satisfaction, remember that
every step you take is a step towards reclaiming
control over your sexual health and well-being. It
takes guts and resolve to address problems like
premature ejaculation, but by taking proactive
steps, you're already on the path to
improvement.

Believe in yourself and your ability to make good
changes. Recognize that success may not always
be straight, but each effort you put in, no matter
how small, adds to your total growth and
development. Celebrate your successes, no
matter how small they may seem, and be gentle
with yourself during failures.

You are not alone in this journey. Lean on your partner for support and understanding, and consider getting advice from healthcare professionals or therapists who specialise in sexual health. Remember that getting help is a sign of strength, not weakness, and there is no shame in valuing your sexual well-being.

Stay loyal to your goals and stay open to trying new strategies and techniques. Keep an open mind and be patient with yourself as you handle this process. With patience, desire, and a positive attitude, you have the power to overcome obstacles and achieve greater happiness in your sexual adventures.

Above all, remember to value self-care and self-compassion along the way. Your road towards better performance and happiness is a testament to your resilience and drive to living a satisfying life. Keep going forward, and know that better days lie ahead.

You hold within you the power to beat premature ejaculation and experience deeply satisfying intimacy. With the right tools, resolve, and willingness to explore, you can discover new levels of pleasure and satisfaction in your sexual adventures.

Believe in your ability to make positive changes and trust that you are capable of transforming obstacles into chances for growth. Embrace each step of your journey with courage and grit, knowing that every effort you make brings you closer to the fulfilling connection you desire.

You are not defined by any limits or setbacks you may meet along the way. Instead, see them as chances to learn, adapt, and grow. With patience, persistence, and a positive mindset, you can develop the confidence and skills needed to handle intimacy with ease and happiness.

Remember, you are worthy of having profound connection and pleasure in your interactions. Trust in yourself, enjoy the trip, and know that you have the strength and perseverance to overcome any hurdles that may arise. Your way to fulfilling intimacy starts with you, and the options are limitless.